# THE ULTIMATE GUIDE TO GETTING INTO PHYSICIAN ASSISTANT SCHOOL

## Notice

Medicine is an ever-changing science. As new research and clinical experience broaden our knowledge, changes in treatment and drug therapy are required. The author and the publisher of this work have checked with sources believed to be reliable in their efforts to provide information that is complete and generally in accord with the standards accepted at the time of publication. However, in view of the possibility of human error or changes in medical sciences, neither the author nor the publisher nor any other party who has been involved in the preparation or publication of this work warrants that the information contained herein is in every respect accurate or complete, and they disclaim all responsibility for any errors or omissions or for the results obtained from use of the information contained in this work. Readers are encouraged to confirm the information contained herein with other sources. For example and in particular, readers are advised to check the product information sheet included in the package of each drug they plan to administer to be certain that the information contained in this work is accurate and that changes have not been made in the recommended dose or in the contraindications for administration. This recommendation is of particular importance in connection with new or infrequently used drugs.

# THE ULTIMATE GUIDE TO GETTING INTO PHYSICIAN ASSISTANT SCHOOL

**FOURTH EDITION**

**Andrew J. Rodican, PA-C**
Associate Medical Director
Medical Weight Loss Centers, LLC
East Haven, Connecticut

New York  Chicago  San Francisco  Athens  London  Madrid  Mexico City
Milan  New Delhi  Singapore  Sydney  Toronto

The Ultimate Guide to Getting into Physician Assistant School, Fourth Edition

1 2 3 4 5 6 7 8 9   LCR   22 21 20 19 18 17

ISBN 978-1-259-85984-7
MHID 1-259-85984-3

This book was set in Sabon LT Std by MPS Limited.
The editors were Susan Barnes and Brian Kearns.
The production supervisor was Catherine Saggese.
Production management was provided by Charu Verma, MPS Limited.

This book is printed on acid-free paper.

Library of Congress Cataloging-in-Publication Data

Names: Rodican, Andrew J., author.
Title: The ultimate guide to getting into physician assistant school / Andrew J. Rodican.
Description: Fourth edition. | New York : McGraw-Hill Education, [2017]
Identifiers: LCCN 2017005429 | ISBN 9781259859847 (paperback : alk. paper) |
    ISBN 1259859843 (paperback : alk. paper)
Subjects: | MESH: Physician Assistants—education | School Admission Criteria
    | Vocational Guidance | United States
Classification: LCC R697.P45 | NLM W 21.5 | DDC 610.73/72069071173—dc23 LC record available
    at https://www.loc.gov/

*This book is dedicated to my father, James A. Rodican, and to my family...*

*My beautiful wife Allison, whom I love with all my heart and who supports me in good times and bad.*

*My son, Eddie, who is currently on his own path to becoming a PA, and has become a kind and compassionate man; my daughter-in-law Lizzie, whom I love dearly, and my granddaughter Lyla, who lights up my heart with pride and joy.*

*My daughter, Nicole, who has worked extremely hard to achieve all her goals in life, and is driven to help as many people as she can in her job as a social worker.*

*My son Andrew, who makes me smile every day and has more energy than should be allowed by law!*

*My little sweetheart Natalie, who warms my heart with her hugs and kisses.*

*And finally, to the friends of Bill, and my closest friends, Ricky and Jimmy. Without them, this book would never have been published.*

**I am truly blessed!**

# Contents

# Foreword

An old friend and colleague of mine a few years ago asked me to write the foreword to the second edition, originally titled, *Getting into the Physician Assistant School of your Choice*, and now I have been asked to write the foreword for the fourth edition. It's been a little over 10 years and the profession has grown to almost 114,000 PAs in the United States. There are more than 200 PA programs in the United States with programs in Canada, the Netherlands, England, Northern Ireland, and Australia. Other European countries and countries in the Middle East are looking into starting PA programs as well. To be honest with you, I never thought the profession would be so successful and expand as much as it has over the past 40 plus years.

What does this mean to you? It means that the PA profession has a bright future, still meeting the health care needs that the United States and the world are faced with today and in the future.

*The Ultimate Guide to Getting into Physician Assistant School* (McGraw-Hill) that my colleague has written will be its fourth edition, and it is still in demand. The author, Andrew (Andy) J. Rodican, PA-C has a unique background: a medical writer with such publications as, "More Questions than Answers: Hepatitis C Virus in the 90s" (Presented at Yale University School of Medicine) and he previously published the "Injury Report," a medical–legal newsletter he developed for workers' compensation issues and personal injury attorneys in the state of Connecticut. He has had numerous experiences in medicine beginning with the Navy as a Medical Corpsman, graduate of Yale University PA program, and a PA in cardiovascular surgery. He was the director of a post cardio-rehab program and a combined weight loss clinic. He has lectured and traveled over the country giving seminars on getting into a PA program, which recently moved to a Webinar format. Andy previously worked at a Yale University affiliated hospital prior to striking out on his own with the cardio-rehab adventure. Today he is in a group practice in the New Haven area.

Books of any nature are only informational! It is the reader who has to take the information and then make it into a game plan. Your game plan should take into consideration your grades, medical experience, where you would like to live, and the cost of your education. Some schools require a GRE; I suggest you take a review course for the GRE. Following these strategies, you will have the makings of a reasonable plan to accomplishing your goal.

Andy's book, *The Ultimate Guide to Getting into Physician Assistant School*, gives you the basics in developing your personal game plan. It tells you how to evaluate a program, what type of applicant they look for, how to prepare for an interview, and yes, how to dress professionally.

I again encourage you and commend you on your quest to join the PA profession. It is a wonderful profession with a bright future. So, take your plan and start, "A journey of 10,000 miles which begins with a first step" (an old Chinese saying). Now do it, take that step! Get the book and work your plan.

**George F. (Rick) Hillegas, Ed D, MPH, PA-C, DFAAPA**
**Dean, School of Physician Assistant Studies**
**South College, Knoxville, TN**

# Introduction

Are you hoping to join one of the hottest career fields in the country and become a physician assistant (PA)? Where are you now in the PA school application process? Worried you're not a competitive applicant? Discouraged you don't know how to stand out from the crowd? Concerned about the investment of time and money?

Whether you're a first-time applicant, or a reapplicant, *The Ultimate Guide to Getting Into Physician Assistant* School provides you with a blueprint to master every step of the application process: deciding if the PA profession is a good match for your career goals, learning to navigate the CASPA application, writing a killer essay, and learning how to ace the PA school interview. This book will help you go from a "vanilla" applicant, to the "perfect applicant" in no time at all.

Welcome to *The Ultimate Guide to Getting Into Physician Assistant School*, 4th Edition. I continue to publish new editions of this book because becoming a PA has changed my life. My hope is that this book will change your life too, as it has for thousands of PA school applicants before you.

Each chapter in this book provides you with short, no nonsense "how to" answers to your questions, tips from my experience on Yale's PA program admissions committee-- and most of all—insider information gained from over twenty years of coaching and helping thousands of PA school applicants get accepted to PA programs from every state in the country.

With your passion, commitment, motivation, and patience, you will soon rise to the top of the applicant pool much faster than if you go it alone. You'll become a much more confident applicant, you'll get more interviews, and you'll be a Physician Assistant Student (PA-S) before you know it. So turn the page and let's get started on your exciting journey.

# [CHAPTER 1]

# So You Want to be a Physician Assistant

First of all, congratulations! By investing in this book, you've just taken your first step toward achieving your goal of becoming a physician assistant (PA) school student. Whether you're a reapplicant to PA school, or a first-time applicant, this book is going to help you get focused and provide you with all of the information you'll need to conquer the PA school application, essay, and interview process. Armed with this information, you will have a wealth of knowledge to help you become the perfect applicant.

No doubt, being a PA will challenge your intelligence, patience, compassion, and prejudices. But the profession will also reward you emotionally and financially. As you learn about the expanding roles of PAs in the health care system, and the continued growth of the profession, you will realize that PAs are an integral part of the future of health care. You are about to embark on a journey that will allow you to enter one of the best professions in the United States, and have a very bright future ahead of you.

In this chapter, I'm going to define the role of the PA, provide information on the history of the PA profession, and discuss the following:

- The definition of a PA
- The evolution of the PA profession
- How PAs are trained
- The future of the PA profession
- Salaries for PAs

- Six reasons to become a PA versus a physician
- The PA scope of practice
- The six things PA programs look for in a competitive applicant

I've personally had a very rewarding career as a PA, and I wouldn't have changed one thing along the way after practicing over two decades. I hope you are excited to begin your own journey, so let's get started.

## WHAT IS A PA?

If you would like the "official" definition of a PA, visit the American Academy of Physician Assistants (AAPA) website at aapa.org. And, while you're on the AAPA website, I strongly recommend that you consider joining as an affiliate member. The AAPA website provides a wealth of information both for PAs and PA school applicants.

In general, PAs are licensed health care professionals who practice medicine under the supervision of a licensed physician. PAs are considered "dependent" practitioners because of this relationship with a supervising physician. PAs practice in all 50 states and also have prescription writing privileges in all 50 states.

PAs work very autonomously in their designated field of practice, although the level of autonomy will vary from practice to practice. Don't expect to follow your supervising physician around by the proverbial "coattails." A physician who knows how to utilize PAs most effectively will expect you to work autonomously within the scope of the practice, carry your own patient load, and utilize your diagnostic and critical thinking skills. In many situations, PAs may not even work in the same physical location as their supervising physician, but they must always remain in telephone contact. Typically, PAs meet with their supervising physician at least once per week.

Some of the duties and responsibilities of the PA include:

- Taking a medical history
- Performing a medical examination
- Ordering diagnostic testing (lab studies, X-rays, MRIs, etc.)
- Formulating a diagnosis and treatment plan
- Writing prescriptions

- Counseling patients
- Discussing preventative medicine
- Performing yearly physical examinations
- Making rounds in various facilities (hospitals, nursing homes, etc.)
- First-assisting in surgery
- Performing minor surgical procedures
- Administering immunizations

An important part of the PAs job description is to work in collaboration with a variety of members of the health care team physicians, nurses, medical assistants, surgeons, phlebotomists, and many other allied health care professionals. The scope of practice of a PA is heavily dependent upon the type of practice the PA works in, state regulations, experience, and comfort level of the supervising physician.

Some benefits that physician assistants enjoy include: a flexible schedule, lateral mobility (being able to move from one specialty to another without any formal training,) and a high patient satisfaction rate. I've personally worked in five different areas of medicine since becoming a PA in 1994, and I owned my own bariatric medicine practice for eight years of those years.

# THE EVOLUTION OF THE PA PROFESSION: FROM PETER THE GREAT TO POSTGRADUATE DEGREES

The PA profession has an amazingly long history. References to various military medical assistants go back as far as 1650 in the Russian army led by Peter the Great. In the World War II era, Dr. Eugene Stead Jr. developed a curriculum model to fast-track the training of physicians in a 3-year time frame.

During the years from 1961 to 1972, the PA concept came more into focus when Dr. Stead established the first PA program at Duke University, in 1967. He used much the same model that he had used to train World War II physicians. He saw the need for midlevel health practitioners to complement the services and skills of the physicians. The need was even more apparent in the remote areas of the United States, where the medical profession historically did not reach out to underserved populations. The opening of more PA programs during the ensuing period prompted the development of the PA professional organization, the American Academy of Physician Assistants (AAPA), in 1968. In 1970, Kaiser Permanente was the first health maintenance organization (HMO) to employ PAs. And in 1971, Montefiore Medical Center established the first postgraduate surgical residency program.

In an effort to maintain consistency throughout PA programs, the American Medical Association's Committee on Allied Health Education and Accreditation developed training program guidelines in 1971 and implemented the program accreditation process. In 1973, the AAPA held its first conference. The first certifying exam was given in 1973, even before the National Commission on Certification of Physician Assistants (NCCPA) had been incorporated, in 1975.

The NCCPA was established to ensure the public that certified PAs meet established criteria and continue to meet those criteria every 6 years by taking a recertification examination. (As of the time of this writing, the recertification process is now 10 years. The first recertification exam was given in 1981. Also, much state legislation has been implemented concerning the practice of PAs and their prescriptive privileges. National legislation also has been implemented to address PA reimbursement. By 1985, the ranks of PAs had grown to more than 10,000 nationally, prompting the development of *National PA Day* in 1987. By 1988, the *Journal of the American Academy of Physician Assistants* (JAAPA) was first published, complementing the field's first official journal publication in 1977, *Health Practitioner* (later called *Physician Assistant*).

In the 10 years after 1990, misconception and prejudices about PA privileges continued to fall away, allowing for an expanded role for PAs. The number of PA programs doubled. Discussion and implementation of master's-level programs began to take place. In 1993, there were 26,400 PAs in existence, but that number grew to 45,000 by 2002. At the end of 2015, that number increased to 108,717 certified PAs (Tables 1.1 and 1.2).

As of 2016, the Physician Assistant Education Association (PAEA) Program Directory lists 234 PA Programs in the United States, including:

- 38 Programs with Provisional Accreditation
- 20 Programs Developing—Not Accredited
- 11 Programs on Probation
- 1 Program on Administrative Probation

**Table 1.1.** Growth of the PA Profession (1980–2016)

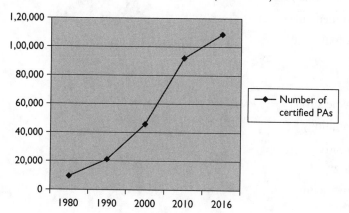

**Table 1.2.** Growth of PA Programs (1980–2016)

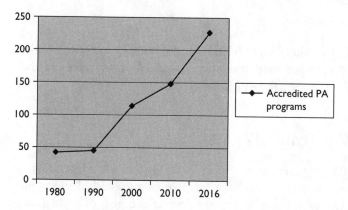

There are also several postgraduate residency programs (Appendix 1) in specialties as diverse as:

- Acute/critical care
- Cardiology
- Cardiothoracic/critical care
- Cardiothoracic surgery
- Child/adolescent psychiatry
- Emergency medicine

- Hematology/oncology
- Hospital medicine
- Neonatology
- Ob-Gyn
- Oncology
- Orthopedic surgery
- Otolaryngology
- Primary care
- Psychology
- Sports medicine
- Surgery
- Surgery/critical care
- Trauma/critical care
- Vascular surgery

The adoption of the PA model in many countries has also resulted in many new PAs. Those internationally trained PAs now represent their home countries at the annual AAPA conference.

## How Are PAs Trained?

The length of PA programs varies from 24 to 32 months, depending on whether the program offers a bachelor's degree or a master's degree. Some programs, like Quinnipiac University in Connecticut, also offer an Entry-Level Master's Physician Assistant Program (ELMPA). The program offers the qualified pre-physician assistant student the opportunity to enter a 4-year pre-professional component and a 27-month professional component. Students can enter this program right out of high school.

PA students are trained in the "medical model," similar to that of most medical schools. In fact, the education process for PAs is often equated to the first 3 years of medical school. Many PA programs are actually affiliated with a medical school and the PA students often share classes with the medical students. The main difference in PA training and physician training is the number of years a physician is required to spend in an internship and residency after the didactic phase of the program is completed.

Students in their first year of a PA program can expect to invest approximately 87 hours per week in the classroom, studying evenings and weekends, and doing some form of volunteer work.

The second year of PA school is dedicated to clinical rotations, where you will work on-site with clinical preceptors at your mandatory and elective clinical rotation sites. Typical mandatory rotations at many programs include:

- Internal Medicine I
- Internal Medicine II
- Primary Care I
- Primary care II
- Emergency Medicine
- General Surgery
- Pediatrics
- Psychiatry
- OB/GYN
- Geriatrics

You will also have the opportunity to select two or three elective rotations in a variety of specialties and clinical rotation sites. The number of hours you work per week on clinical rotations depends on the clinical rotation that you are accomplishing at the time. Psychiatry may be a 9 to 5 schedule, whereas Ob-Gyn may be over 100 hours per week as it was for me.

During clinical rotations you will be assigned a preceptor for the 6- to 12-week rotation, usually a senior resident or a senior PA. You will be assigned your own patients to follow and you will be on a team with other students, interns, and residents. Your job will be to round on your patients every day, check their labs and diagnostic testing results, and be prepared to discuss your findings and proposed treatment plan with the preceptor and the team. You must be prepared on a daily basis, so most students come in very early to read through all of their patient's charts and prepare for getting drilled every morning with questions about your patient's diagnosis and treatment plan by the senior resident or PA.

I personally found that when taking the Physician Assistant National Certification Examination (PANCE) after I graduated, I was able to answer many of the test questions based on my clinical experiences, in addition to my didactic training.

Finally, most of you will be required to complete a master's thesis while on clinical rotations. This could be a collaborative project with other students, and you will also require a great deal of discipline to complete the thesis on time.

## The Future of the PA Profession

To project the future of the PA profession, we must first look at the Association for American Medical Colleges' prediction of a nationwide physician shortage of primary care doctors between "46,000 and 90,000" by 2025.

Between the projected physician shortage and the Affordable Care Act, PAs are in a perfect position to fill this gap. According to the Bureau of Labor Statistics (BLS), the job outlook for PAs from 2014 to 2024 is expected to grow by 30% (much faster than average), with an increase of 28,700 new positions.

NOTE: With the recent election of Donald Trump as the next President, it is safe to say that the Affordable Care Act is likely to become very fluid.

## Salaries for PAs

According to the BLS' Occupational Employment Statistics Survey (2015), the median pay for a PA in the United States is $98,180 per year. There are many PAs who earn in excess of $130,000 per year, and many others who earn $200,000 or more. It all depends on your specialty, number of years' experience, and your negotiating skills.

## Making the Case to Choose a Career as a PA versus MD

I often hear this question from PA school applicants, "Should I become a physician assistant or a physician?" Of course the answer to that question is always a personal one; however, here are six benefits to choosing a career as a PA versus becoming a physician:

1. Physician assistants spend less time in the classroom

   Time to obtain a medical license:

   MD: 9–13 years (counting undergraduate degree)

   PA: 6–7 years (counting undergraduate degree)

2. Becoming a physician assistant is very rewarding

The work environment for PAs is much more suited to their personality. Where MDs and PAs perform the same duties, PAs have a greater focus on patient care. PAs don't need to worry about budgets, billing, collections, and bureaucracy.

PAs also get to feel like part of a team. Physicians are independent practitioners (leaders), who often find themselves running a department or practice.

3. Physician assistants earn a great salary

As mentioned above, the median salary for a PA is over $98,000, and many PAs earn over $130,000 or more. According to the BLS, the median salary for a physician is $187,200 per year. Additionally, because it takes about twice as long to become a physician versus a PA, the loan burden is about double for a physician versus a PA. This translates to PAs having much more net money in their pay checks.

4. Physician assistants have flexible hours

Physicians train to work in one specialty area for their entire career, and are typically locked into that specialty until retirement. If a physician decides to change specialties, he will need to spend several years' additional education and training before making the switch. This also translates to a loss of revenue during that time period.

Once you become a certified physician assistant (PA-C), you already have the training to work in any specialty area of medicine or surgery. That means you can transition from family practice to cardiology without heading back to the classroom or incurring any loss of revenue.

5. Physician assistants work shorter, more regular hours

Physicians not only spend time on patient care, but they must also analyze the practice's revenue and expenditures long after the patients have gone home, and they often work many hours on call.

PAs keep more regular schedules and can choose a position with a lifestyle conducive to their priorities. Once the day is over, the PA gets to go home and spend time pursuing outside interests or with his/her family.

6. Physician assistants have excellent job prospects

In today's environment, a PA can probably quit his job in the morning and have a new one by the afternoon. That might be a stretch, but PAs rarely struggle to find work. Busy physicians are always looking for PAs to extend their practices.

As I mentioned above, job growth for PAs is much higher than the national average (30% by 2022) and even faster than physicians. According to the BLS, job growth for physicians and surgeons is expected to grow by 18% over the same time period.

Becoming a physician is not the only way to enjoy a fulfilling career in medicine. For these reasons, some people find working as a PA more rewarding.

## PAs Scope of Practice

The scope of practice for a PA typically includes diagnosing and prescribing treatment plans for patients, ordering labs and diagnostic testing, prescribing medications, referrals to specialists, and much more. However, each state has its own scope of practice laws for PAs. The following is a great website to see exactly what the scope of practice laws for PAs in any given state may be:

http://www.bartonassociates.com/physician-assistants/physician-assistant-scope-of-practice-laws/

## What Do PA Programs Look for in a Competitive Applicant?

As you'll discover later on in this book, the PA school admissions committee (ADCOM) members already know the qualities that they are looking for in the strongest applicants' way before they even see your CASPA application. Your goal should be to demonstrate to the committee that you have these qualities. Below is a list of what I feel are the most important categories of qualities you will need to demonstrate in order to score the highest with the admissions committee: There are also many more specific qualities that I include under each category listed below.

- Passion for the PA profession
- Academic ability and test scores
- Health care experience

- Understanding of the PA profession
- Maturity
- Ability to handle stress

More on these qualities in the next chapter and the interview chapters.

Okay, so now you know a bit more about the PA profession and you've made your decision to pursue this exciting career path. In the next chapter, we'll take a look at what you'll need to do in order to be the most competitive PA school applicant. I'm going to teach you how to go from being a "Vanilla" applicant, to becoming the "Perfect Applicant."

[CHAPTER 2]

# What Do PA Programs Look for in a Competitive Applicant?

*G*etting accepted to PA school is *extremely* competitive, and it has been for over two decades. You would think that most applicants do their best to meet or exceed all of the minimum requirements to become competitive applicants. I wish this was the case, but after 20 years (to date) of coaching PA school applicants, I can tell you that frequently *is not* the case.

If you frequent the PA Forum (physicianassistantforum.com) as I have, or if you have read the thousands of emails that I have received over the years, you will find that many applicants are looking to get into PA school, skating by with the *minimal* requirements listed on a program's website. These applicants convince themselves that if a PA program requires no medical experience, then there is no need to acquire medical experience. They expect that they will be as competitive as anyone else.

The problem is that over three-quarters of "accepted" PA school applicants come into the application process with prior medical experience (more on this later in the chapter). So although a program doesn't require medical experience, you won't be very competitive without it.

Don't believe me? Let's take a look at the key qualities most PA programs look for in the strongest applicants, and consider the published data (below) as they relate to "accepted" students. The five key qualities include: passion, academic experience and test scores, medical experience, understanding of the PA profession, and maturity.

## Passion

Passion is the rocket fuel that can propel an otherwise-average candidate to the top of the applicant pool. Passion is the burning desire that motivates the perfect applicant to study that extra hour, take that extra chemistry course, repeat classes where she's done poorly, or gain that extra year of hands-on medical experience *before* applying to PA school. Passion takes the words *I can't*, and replaces them with, *I will*. Passion cannot be taught; it must come from deep within.

Unfortunately, too many applicants want to cut corners because of their desire to apply to PA school now! These applicants do not want to do the *work* necessary to become a competitive applicant as demonstrated in the data included in Tables 2.1 to 2.4.

If you truly have the passion for becoming a PA, you will take certain steps, and do the work necessary to be most competitive. Here are 10 steps successful PA school applicants will take to become the perfect applicant:

> STEP 1: Take an extra year to strengthen their application (if necessary.)
>
> STEP 2: Accomplish *all* of the prerequisites needed to become a competitive applicant at the school(s) in which they choose to apply.
>
> STEP 3: Find a way to gain another year of medical experience if needed.
>
> STEP 4: Retake extra science courses, or those science courses where they did not receive a competitive grade.
>
> STEP 5: Join the AAPA.
>
> STEP 6: Join their constituent/state chapter of the AAPA.
>
> STEP 7: Find four PAs to shadow.
>
> STEP 8: Do their homework on the programs where they plan to apply. (More on how to do this in the interview chapters.)
>
> STEP 9: Learn to write a *killer* essay; have it reviewed and edited before submitting it.
>
> STEP 10: Review interview questions and answers, and practice by doing a mock interview before the big day.

Remember, there is no easy way, or short-cut, to get into PA school. You must *do the work* and earn your seat in a program.

A key benefit of having passion is the motivation it provides. On Saturday nights, when you would prefer to be out with your friends rather than studying pharmacology or microbiology, your passion will keep you focused. On clinical rotations, when you are spending your nights in the on-call room at the hospital, rather than sleeping in your own bed, it is your passion for becoming a PA that will make it all seem worthwhile.

**Exercise**

List five things you've done to demonstrate your passion for becoming a PA. Examples might include shadowing experiences, medical experience, taking additional science courses to raise your GPA or to make up for a poor grade, becoming a member of the American Academy of Physician Assistants (AAPA) and your state/constituent chapter of the AAPA.

1. _____
   _____

2. _____
   _____

3. _____
   _____

4. _____
   _____

5. _____
   _____

# Academic Ability and Test Scores

When reviewing your application, the admissions committee will consider two key factors:

1. Do you have the academic ability to complete a rigorous didactic program?
2. If you complete the program, will you be able to pass your boards?

There is no absolute way to answer these questions with 100% certainty. However, you should be aware of the average GPA and GRE scores of *accepted* students as reported in the *Thirtieth* (2015) *Annual Report on Physician Assistant Educational Programs in the United States.* This report is published annually and can be found on the Physician Assistant Education Association's (PAEA's) website (paeaonline.org). These data are current as of 2015, and represent the actual data of applicants who are currently in their first year of PA school.

**Table 2.1.** First-Year Class: Grade Point Averages

| GPA Category | M | SD | Mdn | n(P) |
|---|---|---|---|---|
| Overall undergraduate: | 3.52 | 0.14 | 3.52 | 176 |
| Undergraduate science | 3.47 | 0.16 | 3.49 | 163 |
| CASPA biology, chemistry, physics (BCP) | 3.42 | 0.17 | 3.45 | 84 |
| Undergraduate non-science | 3.54 | 0.20 | 3.59 | 88 |

**Table 2.2.** First-Year Class GRE Scores

| GRE Scores | M | SD | Mdn | n(P) |
|---|---|---|---|---|
| Verbal reasoning: | 152.2 | 5.32 | 153 | 59 |
| Quantitative reasoning | 152 | 3.68 | 152 | 55 |
| Analytical writing | 3.9 | 0.28 | 4.0 | 50 |

Exercise

Fill in the blanks and compare your data to the data above.

**Table 2.3.** My GPA

| GPA Category |
|---|
| Overall undergraduate: |
| Undergraduate science |
| CASPA biology, chemistry, physics (BCP) |
| Undergraduate non-science |

**Table 2.4.** My GRE Scores

| GRE Scores |
| --- |
| Verbal reasoning: |
| Quantitative reasoning |
| Analytical writing |

How do your GPA and GRE scores compare with former, first-year, accepted students? Are you a competitive applicant?

Are you now feeling depressed? Hopeless? Don't worry, the good news is that Admissions Committees (ADCOMs) will also consider *trends* rather than absolute numbers. For instance, if your GPA is 3.1, but your last ten hard science courses were all A's, you show an upward trend. The committee may take this into consideration when reviewing your application and deciding if you can handle graduate-level science coursework. This is why I always recommend retaking science classes where you may have done poorly.

Let's look at a hypothetical example of what I'm talking about in Table 2.5, comparing Mary's trend to Bob's trend.

**Table 2.5.** Grade Trends

| Year in School | Mary | | Bob | |
| --- | --- | --- | --- | --- |
| Freshman | General Chemistry: | D | General Chemistry: | A |
| | Microbiology: | C | Microbiology: | A |
| Sophomore | Organic Chemistry I: | C | Organic Chemistry I: | A |
| | Biochemistry I: | B | Biochemistry I: | B |
| Junior | Inorganic Chemistry: | A | Inorganic Chemistry: | C |
| | Organic Chemistry II: | A | Organic Chemistry II: | C |
| Senior | Physical Chemistry: | A | Physical Chemistry: | C |
| | Genetics: | A | Genetics: | D |

In the above table we can see that both Mary and Bob have a 3.0 GPA. Mary's trend is upward and Bob's trend is downward, as evidenced by the above data for each successive year in undergraduate school.

If both Mary and Bob were to take five or six post-graduate science courses, or retake the courses where they've done poorly, they can also demonstrate an upward trend and possibly convince the admissions committee that they can do the work, especially if they have a strong application otherwise.

Additionally, remember that *median* scores mean that half of the applicant's GPAs are above the median score, and half of the applicant's GPAs are below the median score. So if you're GPA is slightly below the mean GPA for accepted students, don't despair.

Here are some other things the ADCOM will consider.

## Number of Credit Hours per Semester

A typical day in PA school requires students to sit in a classroom for 8 to 10 hours per day, perhaps spend an early evening physical examination seminar, and then study for three or four hours afterward in preparation for a pharmacology exam the next day. This rigorous daily schedule demands excellent time-management skills, as well as the ability to comprehend and assimilate large volumes of scientific material. The only means in which ADCOMs have to evaluate whether you can make the grade in this area is by reviewing your transcripts. Applicants who carried a full course load, played a sport, and worked part-time will likely make a more favorable impression with the committee than an applicant who took fewer classes and did not participate in any extracurricular activities.

## Course Difficulty

The admissions committee will more likely favor an applicant who was a chemistry major with a 3.2 GPA, versus an applicant who was a history major with a GPA of 3.4. Remember, the ADCOM is looking for applicants who will thrive while accomplishing graduate-level science coursework.

## Reputation of the College/University

Although the interpretation of GPAs from an Ivy League school versus a State University can be very subjective, I think you would agree that a

3.3 GPA from Harvard would trump a 3.6 GPA from a State University. I only mention this because many applicants will take several classes at a community college and think an "A" is an "A," but it doesn't necessarily work that way.

## Life Difficulties and Circumstances

We all experience challenges and difficulties in the course of our lives, some more than others. The ADCOM will take these challenges into consideration when reviewing your application, especially if you have a lower GPA than most. Some significant stressors include divorce, death of a parent/sibling/spouse, or a serious medical illness. Your job is to demonstrate how you've overcome these challenges and how you've become a stronger person as a result of going through the pain. Don't make excuses or expect pity. Being genuine and honest will go a long way toward making your case.

## Extracurricular Activities

Your GPA and GRE scores aren't everything when it comes to the admission process. ADCOMs are seeking well-rounded individuals with real-life experiences. I've read thousands of PA school applications, and when I see that someone has been in the military, played a sport in college, or even worked for the Peace Corps, I automatically reflect on the *inherent* qualities this person has that will make him a great student and a great PA.

If an applicant has been in the military, I automatically think of the following qualities:

- discipline
- attention to detail
- leadership
- teamwork

An applicant who played a college-level sport demonstrates:

- the ability to multi-task (travel, practice, and perform well in the classroom)
- teamwork
- discipline

Someone who has worked in the Peace Corps would tend to be:

- selfless
- compassionate
- empathetic

Think about any extracurricular activities that pertain to you, and be sure to mention them in your essay or at your interview.

## Standardized Test Scores

Most programs require GRE scores, and the median scores are listed above. However, while on the admissions committee at Yale, I found that test scores did not play a significant role in the decision process. If you have a 3.7 GPA in chemistry, 10 years of medical experience, and 3,000 hours of volunteer work, I could care less if your GRE scores are a little low. Many people simply do not do well on standardized tests.

This is strictly my opinion and how I weighed test scores when I was on the admissions committee at Yale. You should be aware, however, that there are a few schools that *do* have an absolute requirement for GRE scores. I don't agree with this philosophy, but you must take it into consideration if you are applying to one of these programs. Thankfully, these programs are the exception and not the rule!

# Medical Experience

I've always been amazed by the fact that young students coming right out of college with no prior medical experience definitively know that they want to become physicians and attend medical school. I think the fact that most applicants accepted to PA school have over 2,000 hours of patient contact experience is a tribute to the PA profession. It is also a reason why those applicants with little or no medical experience are far less competitive than those who have accumulated hours.

Unlike applying to medical school, PA school applicants need to gain some form of medical experience prior to applying. Tables 2.6 to 2.9 list data relative to various types of medical experience and the mean number of hours of medical experience for students accepted into PA programs.

**Table 2.6.** Medical Experience Statistics for PA School Applicants

| | |
|---|---|
| Worked in health care before applying to PA school | 79% |
| Worked less than one year or not at all in a health care field | 27% |
| Worked more than nine years in a health care field | 10% |
| Worked less than one year or not at all in a health care field with direct patient contact | 35% |
| Previously worked as a medical assistant | 17% |
| Previously worked as an EMT/Paramedic | 9% |
| Worked as a phlebotomist | 9% |
| Worked as an emergency room technician | 8% |
| Worked in medical reception/records | 7% |
| Worked as a nurse | 8% |
| Worked as an athletic trainer | 6% |
| Reported "other" as health care experience | 45% |

Note: Respondents were permitted to indicate multiple health care fields; thus, the sum of all fields exceeds 100%.

**Table 2.7.** Average Health Care Experience Hours of Matriculating Students

| Health Care Experience | M | SD | Mdn | n(P) |
|---|---|---|---|---|
| Patient contact experience | 3,100 | 3,006 | 2,325 | 89 |
| Other health care experience | 1,014 | 943 | 713 | 30 |
| Other work experience | 2,001 | 1,771 | 1,500 | 21 |
| Community service | 425 | 480 | 270 | 32 |
| Shadowing | 144 | 204 | 88 | 45 |

**Exercise**

Fill in the blanks to see how you compare with accepted students.

**Table 2.8.** My Health Care Experience Hours

| Health Care Experience | # Hours |
|---|---|
| Patient contact experience | |
| Other health care experience | |
| Other work experience | |
| Community service | |
| Shadowing | |

Hopefully, now you will have a much better understanding of why I stress the importance of having medical experience prior to applying to PA school.

# Understanding of the PA Profession

The PA profession is growing by leaps and bounds and is projected to be one of the top professions for job growth in the future. The salaries are excellent and jobs are plentiful. Because of this favorable outlook, some applicants who apply to PA school are just *testing the waters*, or throwing their hat in the ring to see if they can pull off getting accepted into this phenomenal career field. ADCOMs can usually spot these applicants a mile away. These applicants don't have a thorough understanding of the PA profession because they're not in it for the right reasons. This is why it is so important to understand the role of the PA and convince the ADCOM that you genuinely want to become a PA for the right reasons.

Therefore, if you plan on applying to PA school, it is imperative that you do the work and develop a strong understanding of the role of PAs in our health care system. You should also know about current events as well as *hot topics* in the news.

The best way to learn about the role of the PA is to shadow PAs. Shadow PAs in various specialties and observe their roles in different clinical settings. Ask a lot of questions and take notes. Become aware of the challenges PAs face on a daily basis. Ask the PAs you shadow what they like and don't like about being a PA. Make sure you walk away from these experiences with a thorough understanding of the PA profession.

The best way to stay current with the PA profession, and to learn about hot topics in the news, is to join the AAPA and your state/constituent chapter of the AAPA. Everything you need to know about the PA profession: current events, hot topics, and PA legislation can be found on these websites. Additionally, if you join these organizations you will receive a monthly journal (*The Journal of the American Academy of Physician Assistant*) and a monthly, or quarterly, newsletter from your state chapter.

You will not regret the modest investment it takes to join these organizations, and you will be way ahead of most of the competition if you do so.

Foreign Medical Graduates (FMGs) receive far more scrutiny than typical applicants. As a result, FMGs must be able to articulate that they have a thorough understanding of the PA profession, and must be able to convince the ADCOM that they are fully aware of the dependent (italics) nature of the profession.

Some key questions the admissions committee considers concerning FMGs include:

1. Are you going to be able to adapt to the role of a *dependent* practitioner?
2. Are you using PA school as a stepping-stone to gain access to medical school in the United States?

Let's now examine 10 common questions that you will likely be asked relative to your understanding of the PA profession:

1. Why do you want to be a PA?
2. What are some of the challenges facing the PA profession?
3. Tell us about some current events relative to the PA profession.
4. What are some hot topics in the news right now concerning PAs?
5. If you could change one thing about the PA profession, what would that be?
6. What is a *dependent* practitioner?

7. How do PAs differ from MDs?
8. What's the difference between a nurse practitioner and a PA?
9. Why don't you want to become a physician?
10. How many PAs have you shadowed?

In the interview chapters, I cover answers to many of these questions. But it is your job to do the work, and develop a comprehensive understanding of the PA profession through the ways I discussed above.

## Maturity

Although maturity isn't only defined by age, it is a fact that the mean age of a first-year PA student is 26 years. Having said that, I have personally interviewed thousands of younger applicants who display a high level of maturity, even at the age of 21. These applicants have a diverse background, a good deal of medical experience, and the ability to present themselves in a professional manner.

**Table 2.9.** Age-Related Statistics

| First-Year Class: Age | M | SD | Mdn | n(P) |
|---|---|---|---|---|
| Age of first-year PA student | 26.1 | 2.51 | 26.0 | 170 |
| Age of youngest first-year PA student | 21.4 | 1.23 | 21.0 | 168 |
| Age of oldest first-year PA student | 44.1 | 7.57 | 44.0 | 168 |

When I do a mock interview with an applicant, I subconsciously ask myself this question: Would I want this person taking care of my daughter in the emergency room or ICU?

So how does an applicant demonstrate maturity in an interview? Mature applicants exhibit the following traits:

- They know how to be empathetic, yet assertive.
- They can handle stress under fire.
- They know when to call for help.
- They exhibit good judgment.

- They can make quick decisions.
- They are self-aware.
- They are self-starters.
- They won't require constant supervision.
- They don't make excuses for their shortcomings.

The best PA school applicants come from diverse backgrounds and possess a variety of life experiences. Some of the most interesting candidates have careers that are totally unrelated to health care at the time of the application. However, these applicants have demonstrated the qualities that PA programs look for in the perfect applicant (more on this in the interview chapters).

Now that you have an understanding of the specific traits the ADCOM looks for in strong applicants, let's see if we can come up with your personalized plan to achieve this worthy goal.

# CHAPTER 3

# Your PAth to Success: Setting Goals

*Whatever the mind of man can conceive and believe, it can achieve.*

—Napolean Hill (Author, *Think and Grow Rich*)

I believe we all have goals in life, but how many of us actually have a plan to carry them out? Goals must be specific, have a deadline for achievement, and must be committed to writing in order to have the best chance of being realized.

At the age of 16, I had two main goals in life: to become an entrepreneur and to work in medicine. One may think these goals required separate paths in life; however, as you will see, I would ultimately achieve both of these goals. In this chapter I hope to help you achieve your goal to become a PA, and I will show you exactly how you can develop your personalized plan to do so.

## WHY SET GOALS?

Few people ever bother to set realistic goals in life. Most people are what the famous author and motivational speaker, Zig Ziglar, calls "wandering generalit[ies]" but need to become "meaningful specific[s]." The bottom line is that the competition for admission to PA school is fierce. Without a written goal, a plan of action, and the ability to have a razor-like focus, your chances of being accepted to the program of your choice are slim.

The basic problem most people have with setting goals is not time, it's a lack of direction. We all have the same 24 hours in each day. Why is it some people achieve so much, while others who are equally as intelligent and capable cannot seem to accomplish anything? Because the former have goals—written, measurable, and realistic goals—and they know how to achieve them. Numerous authors, from Stephen Covey to Norman Vincent Peale, have discussed how to go about setting goals. They both agree: having specific long-term and short-term goals will lead you to become more creative, which will, in turn, add more excitement and fulfillment to your life.

Do you know why 97% of people never really set goals in the proper fashion? As Zig Ziglar says, the answer is fear, or *false evidence appearing real.* But what are we afraid of? Some of us are afraid of failure. Some of us fear the competition. Some of us are actually afraid of success. After all, there is danger in setting goals—we might actually achieve them! We've all heard the phrase, *be careful what you wish for.*

But I propose to you that there is more danger in not setting goals, especially the danger of wasting your resources. As they say, a boat in dry dock rots more quickly than a boat at sea. Don't waste *your* resources, and write down your goals today!

If I haven't convinced you of the importance of goal setting yet, perhaps this next story will.

In 1953, a study at Yale University polled graduating seniors about how many of them had written goals and a plan of action for carrying them out. Here are the results of that study:

- Three percent had a complete plan.
- Ten percent had taken some steps.
- Eighty-seven percent had set no goals at all and had no plan of action for life after graduation: wandering generalities!

In 1973, twenty years later, the university polled those same seniors again. This time, researchers asked them about their successes in measurable areas: finances, career, and position in life. Not surprisingly, the 3% of graduates, who had set goals and developed a written plan of action to carry them out, had accomplished more than the other 97% combined.

## SEVEN-STEP FORMULA FOR SUCCESS

If you utilize the following seven-step formula for success, you too will be able to accomplish *any* worthy goal in life. Follow these simple steps to maximize your chances of getting into the PA school of your choice:

1. Identify the goal.
2. Set a deadline for achievement.
3. List obstacles to overcome.
4. Identify people and organizations that can help you.
5. List the skills and knowledge required to achieve the goal.
6. Develop a plan of action.
7. List the benefits of achieving the goal, and ask yourself: *What's in it for me?*

Now, take out a piece of paper and begin listing your goals. If you do nothing else with this book, you will at least have completed your personalized goal sheet by the end of this chapter. If you need some help getting started, let's take a look at my personal goal statement from 1992. You'll notice I wrote mine out in paragraph format, but you may commit your goals to writing in any format you desire. The point is to get started and get it done; sooner rather than later!

August 15, 1990

By May 1, 1992 I will be accepted into one, or all, of the following PA programs: Yale, Florida, or Wake Forest (Bowman Gray.) To accomplish this goal, I first have to discuss my desire to become a PA with my wife and convince her that this is the right thing to do for our family. Next, I need to begin saving money so that I can help my wife support our two children and provide food and shelter for the next 2 years. Finally, I will stay focused and not listen to those people who will say, "You're crazy for doing this, are you having a mid-life crisis? You are thirty-five years old, have a great job, and will have to give that up to go to school for two years."

I will immediately contact the American Academy of Physician Assistants (AAPA) and the Connecticut Academy of Physician Assistants (ConnAPA) to sign up for an affiliate membership and find out what resources are available to me. I will order a copy of the PA Programs Directory (now available online) and begin writing to several schools, focusing on my three top choices. I will contact the president of ConnAPA and get to know him. I will also visit Yale's PA program and visit with Elaine Grant, the dean of the program, and maintain contact with her quarterly. I will also correspond with my two top choice programs quarterly. I will inquire from each program about my strengths and weaknesses and learn what I can do to become a stronger applicant.

I will shadow several PAs who work in the multi-specialty practice where my wife works. I will attend as many Open Houses as possible to learn more about the program, have discussions with the students, and learn more about the culture of the program.

I will take courses in Anatomy & Physiology (I & II) and microbiology to fulfill prerequisite requirements. I will achieve no less than an A in each class. I will also begin volunteering at Saint Raphael's hospital emergency room, to gain more current patient contact hours. I will also purchase a SAT study guide and prepare myself to score high on the SATs, which are needed to apply to Yale's PA program.

My plan is to continue working full-time, save money, and do volunteer work part-time. I will also take the prerequisite classes in the evening. While volunteering in the hospital, I will discuss my goal with as many PAs as possible, and learn as much as I can about the PA profession and the scope of practice in each specialty.

Once I achieve my goal of getting into the PA school of my choice, I will enjoy many benefits: helping people, job satisfaction, a secure future, challenging and stimulating work, prestige, a sense of accomplishment, and earning a great salary.

Fast-forward to 2016. I am in my 24th year of clinical practice as a Yale graduate PA. I have worked in five different areas of medicine, including owning my own medical weight loss practice for 8 years. Deciding to become a PA was one of the best choices I have made in my life. I never regretted it for one instant. If I listened to those saboteurs who advised me not to give up my job when I was applying, I would have never experienced the challenges and opportunities that I have had as a PA. By the way, the monetary investment paid off significantly.

### Exercise

Before completing this chapter, I would like you to accomplish writing your own personal goal sheet for getting accepted to PA school. The first thing you will need to do before getting started is to select at least five programs that you want to attend. You can certainly add more programs if you like. Keep in mind that we will discuss selecting programs in the next chapter, so you can always come back to this later.

### List your top five PA programs

1. _____

2. _____

3. _____

4. _____

5. _____

**[Steps 1 and 2] Identify your goal and set a deadline for achievement**

I will be accepted to the _____PA
program by _____, 20___.

**[Step 3] List obstacles to overcome**

- _____
- _____
- _____
- _____
- _____
- _____
- _____
- _____
- _____
- _____

**[Step 4] Identify people and organizations that can help you**

A few examples are listed below to get you started:

a) AJR Associates (Andy Rodican-PA-C @ andrewrodican.com)
b) The American Academy of Physician Assistants (AAPA)
c) State/constituent chapter of the AAPA
d)
e)
f)

**[Step 5] List the skills and knowledge required to achieve your goal**

a) Gain 1,000 more hours of patient contact
b) Take microbiology and organic chemistry 2

c) _____

d) _____

e) _____

f) _____

g) _____

h) _____

i) _____

j) _____

## [Step 6] Develop a plan of action

_____

_____

_____

_____

_____

_____

_____

_____

_____

## [Step 7] List the benefits of achieving the goal, and ask yourself: *What's in it for me? What's the payoff?*

A few examples are listed below:

a) Excellent job-growth potential

b) Job satisfaction

c) _____

d) _____

e) _____

f) _____

g) _____

h) _____

i) _____

Now it's time to officially write out your personalized goal sheet. Be as specific as possible, laminate the sheet, and put it in a place where you will see it, and read it, every day.

Date: __/__/____

_____

_____

_____

_____

_____

## IMAGING

Setting goals and committing them to writing is a powerful way to succeed at anything in life. However, I want to mention a technique that most professional athletes and successful people all over the world use to magnify their chances of achieving goals. The technique is called *imaging*.

The epigraph to this chapter—*Whatever the mind of man can conceive and believe, it can achieve*—is what first sparked my interest in using imaging as a tool to reach my goals. Let me share with you how I used this technique to help me get accepted to Yale's PA program:

> When I decided to apply to PA school, I immediately developed my goal sheet and decided to incorporate imaging into my daily routine. While visiting the Yale PA program one day, I asked for an envelope with the program's logo on it. I placed that envelope against the side of my television. Every day I would work out in my bedroom on an old NordicTrack ski machine. During that entire work out, I would stare at that envelope with the Yale PA school logo, and picture myself walking out to my mail box, seeing the envelope, opening it, and reading, "Congratulations . . ."
>
> As I did this each and every day, my heart rate would actually increase and my breathing would become rapid and shallow, as if I were really walking to the mail box and seeing the letter inside. I calculated that I used this technique for almost 200 hours by the time I actually did receive that acceptance letter.

This technique worked for me and I am confident it will work for you too.

Another tool you can use to *supercharge* your motivation, and enhance your chances of achieving your goal, is to create a *vision board*. I learned about this technique after reading a best-selling 2006 self-help book titled, *The Secret*. Written by Rhonda Byrne, this book is based on the law of attraction and claims that positive thinking can create life-changing results such as increased happiness, health, and wealth.

In *The Secret*, one of the contributors mentions using a vision board as a tool to fulfill your goals. A vision board can be made by taking a blank poster board and placing a variety of pictures, logos, and any visual material that you can see on a daily basis to remind yourself of what you want to achieve in your life.

For instance, if you want to attend Baylor's PA program, you might add:

- pictures of the PA school building
- pictures of Baylor PA students in the classroom
- Baylor PA program logo/letterhead
- pictures of PAs in clinical practice
- pictures of Baylor PA students graduating
- a typed letter (written by yourself) on Baylor letterhead reading: *Dear John. Congratulations, you've been accepted into the Baylor PA program's upcoming class...*

You can do this for any/all of the programs where you wish to attend. Looking at these pictures on a daily basis will give the message to your subconscious brain that this is your chief goal right now, and your subconscious brain will go to work for you trying to make this happen.

## TAKE A PERSONAL INVENTORY

In addition to creating your goal sheet and making a vision board, I also recommend that you review your qualifications and evaluate those areas in which you need improvement. Going to PA school will be a major transition, and before you jump in head first you will need to take a personal inventory. The best way to approach this personal inventory is to evaluate seven specific areas in your life.

I like to use the analogy of spokes on wheel. If the spokes are all the same size, the wheel will ride nice and smoothly. However, if some of the spokes are short and some are long, you're going to have a bumpy ride.

The purpose of the personal inventory is to balance out your life so that it will run smoothly.

Periodically, evaluate yourself in the following seven areas:

1. <u>Appearance</u>: Do I present myself well? Do I need to lose some weight or buy a new pair of shoes before the interview?

2. <u>Family</u>: Is my family supportive of my goal? Will this career change cause conflict in my family life? Am I willing to ignore the skeptics and follow my dream unconditionally?

3. <u>Financial</u>: Can I afford to attend PA school now? Can I afford *not* to go to PA school now? Will I be able to obtain student loans? Can I save enough money to make the financial burden less stressful?

4. <u>Social</u>: Am I a team player? Will I make a good classmate? What do I have to offer? Am I willing to practice medicine as a dependent practitioner?

5. <u>Spiritual</u>: Is it morally right to become a PA at this time? Am I choosing this profession for the right reasons? Am I being selfish to my family?

6. <u>Mental</u>: Do I need to take additional courses, or retake some courses? Am I well-read on the PA profession? Will I have too many distractions?

7. <u>Career</u>: Do I have a thorough understanding of why I want to become a PA versus a nurse practitioner or a physician? Do I fully understand the role of a PA?

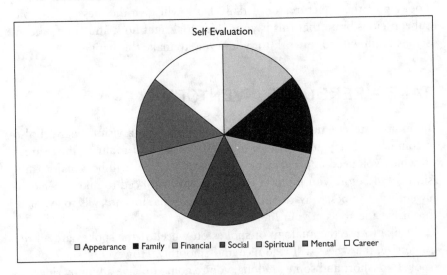

How do your spokes look? Score your answers on a scale from 1 to 5, with 5 being the highest and 1 being the lowest. Be honest with yourself. Is your life balanced in these seven areas? Where can you improve? By taking this personal inventory, you will be able to focus in on areas where you're deficient and make the necessary changes to reach your goal of becoming a PA.

## SET BIG GOALS

*I bargained with Life for a Penney,*
*And Life would pay no more;*
*However, I begged at evening*
*When I counted my scanty store.*

*For Life is a just employer;*
*He gives you what you ask,*
*But once you have set the wages,*
*Why, you must bear the task.*

*I worked for a menial's hire,*
*Only to learn, dismayed,*
*That any wage I had asked of Life,*
*Life would have willingly paid.*

**—Jesse B. Rittenhouse**

Here's a quick story to drive home the point of setting big goals.

As the story goes, there were two men fishing on a pier, one older and one younger. The young man watched as the older man kept reeling in big fish, but throwing them back into the water.

Being curious, the young man asked: *Why are you throwing back those big, beautiful fish? Because I only have this small frying pan,* responded the older man, as he held up his tiny skillet.

Without setting big goals, you will never accomplish big things! The old fisherman was a great fisherman, but his skillet—his goal—was too small. Dig down deep into your soul and focus on what you want in life. Make a plan and envision yourself accomplishing each task. Ralph Waldo Emerson once wrote: *What lies behind us and what lies before us are tiny matters compared to what lies within us.*

## WITH WHOM DO I SHARE MY GOALS?

Some goals we set are "give-up" goals, designed to let go or get rid of something. For example, if you set a goal to lose 20 pounds of body weight (give-up goal), then let everybody in the office, your family, and your friends know about it.

In contrast, a "go-up" goal is designed to get you something: a new job, more financial security, an invitation to join a PA program. Share go-up goals only with your closest friends and family members, as they are the ones most likely to support you. The last thing you need when trying to achieve a go-up goal is to share your goal with a saboteur.

## GETTING FOCUSED

I'd like to touch on the power of focus. Just because you've decided to apply to PA school, does not mean that *life* stops happening. You will still need to deal with the daily stressors that life throws your way, like finding the time to research schools, completing the CASPA application, working full-time, taking classes in the evening, and managing financial pressures. Some of you may find it overwhelming to deal with all of these issues, and perhaps want to throw in the towel. Don't worry, you're not alone! Everyone feels this way at one point or another during the PA school application process. When you feel this way, remember this one saying: *Obstacles are those frightful things we see when we take our eyes off our goal.* Stay focused!

## THE TOURNAMENT DRAW TECHNIQUE

Because you will have many items on your "to-do" list, I am going to share with you a great technique to get organized, and also help you accomplish those mini-goals that you will need to complete on your way to your primary goal: getting accepted to PA school.

The number of items you will need to accomplish can seem a bit overwhelming, and this technique is meant to help you prioritize them by importance.

This technique is patterned after the "March Madness" NCAA basketball tournament brackets. At the beginning of the tournament, the brackets are posted in each division, and those who win continue to progress to the next round. Eventually, we end up with the "sweet sixteen," the "elite eight," the "final four," and finally the championship game between the last two teams standing. The winner of the championship game ultimately becomes the NCAA champion.

The following diagram is patterned after this technique, and instead of placing teams in the brackets, you will place the items you need to accomplish before selecting a program and accomplishing the CASPA application.

Let's take a look at some of those things you may need to accomplish in order to apply to PA school:

1. Take the GREs
2. Complete prerequisite microbiology course
3. Shadow one more PA
4. Secure one more person to write a LOR
5. Write the essay
6. Gain 500 more hours of medical experience
7. Complete the CASPA application
8. Attend "open houses" at top-choice schools

Not let's put these items into the tournament draw bracket. Just list them on the left side of the bracket in no particular order. Compare each pair of items (#1 with #2) and decide which one is more important, then advance that item to "Round 2." Do the same for items #3 and #4, #5 and #6, and #7 and #8. The point is to keep advancing the most important items to Round 2, then repeat the comparisons until you have a "winner," or the priority you will need to accomplish on your "to-do" list.

I am going to use 8 items in this example, but this technique will work for 16 items, 24 items, or however many items you have.

So, let's look at the hypothetical list above and place them into Round 1 of the "Tournament Draw Technique" (Table 3.1).

In the example above, here is my rationale for making my choices; your choices certainly may be different. I compared #1 with #2 in Round 1, and decided it was more important to complete the prerequisite microbiology class before taking the GRE. Without the microbiology class, I would not meet all of the prerequisites of the program and I would be ineligible to apply. I could always take the GREs later, even concurrently with** the microbiology course. The microbiology class, therefore, moves on to Round 2.

Then I compared #3 with #4 in Round 1, and I decided it is more important to find another PA to shadow before securing another person to write my letter of recommendation. Although both may be equally import-ant, I believe it will be harder to find a PA to shadow and accumulate

**Table 3.1.** The Tournament Draw Technique Format

| Round 1 | Round 2 | Round 3 | Winner |
|---------|---------|---------|--------|
| 1. Take GREs | Microbiology | | |
| 2. Take microbiology | | Microbiology | |
| 3. Shadow PA | Shadow | | Microbiology |
| 4. LOR | | | |
| 5. Write essay | Medical experience | | |
| 6. Medical experience | | Medical experience | |
| 7. Complete CASPA | Attend open house | | |
| 8. Attend open house | | | |

40

hours with that person, than securing another person to write my letter of recommendation. I may even be able to have the PA I shadow write a LOR for me. Shadowing another PA moves on to Round 2.

Next I compared #5 with #6 in Round 1, and I decided that I need to gain 500 more hours of medical experience to be most competitive. I could write the essay while accumulating those hours. Therefore, gaining 500 hours of medical experience moves on to Round 2.

Finally, I compared #7 with #8 in Round 1, and decided it would be better to attend the program's open house before accomplishing the CASPA application. I will probably learn a lot about the program at the open house, and have an opportunity to meet with students of the program. The information I learn at the open house will be beneficial to me when writing my essay and answering questions at the interview. Attending the open house moves on to Round 2.

The process continues by deciding which items move on to the third round, and ultimately the winner. In the above example, taking the prerequisite microbiology course is the winner, and would be my number one priority. I can now work backwards (Round 3 to Round 1) and continue to accomplish my priorities that are now listed in each bracket. For instance, my next goal would be to go back to Round 3, and realize my next goal is to gain 500 hours of additional medical experience. I could also do this part-time while completing the microbiology course. Keep moving backwards in the rounds until you are finished. Okay, so now that you've joined the top 3% of achievers by writing down your goals, it's time to take a look at the multitude of PA programs and decide which programs will be the best "fit" for your qualifications. This will be an exciting process, but you must do your homework!

See Appendix 2 for a blank Tournament Draw Technique format that you can accomplish using your own to-do list. Remember, you can expand the list, and the chart, to add additional items.

# [CHAPTER 4]

# Selecting a PA Program

The excitement is starting to build. You've made the commitment to apply to PA school, you have a written goal, and your next task is to select the program(s) that you want to attend. At the time of this writing, there are over 234 programs to choose from. You may be a bit overwhelmed at this point, but I want you to realize that you should have a common denominator for all of the programs you select. Ask yourself, why am I applying to these particular programs, versus any other programs?

Here is an actual question that one of my coaching applicants was asked at her PA school interview:

> "Provide us with a list of all the schools you've applied to, why you applied there, which are your top schools and why, where you received interviews, and which is your first choice?"

Wow, what a question! Not every program is going to ask you this question, but you should at least be prepared to answer what your rationale is for applying to the programs you've chosen.

## A FEW QUESTIONS TO CONSIDER BEFORE SELECTING YOUR PROGRAM(S)

1. Is the program accredited by the Accreditation Review Commission on Education for the Physician Assistant (ARC-PA?)

   ARC-PA is the accrediting agency that defines the standards for PA education and evaluating PA educational programs within the territorial United States to ensure their compliance with those standards.

The very first criteria you should look for in a PA program you're considering is its accreditation status. The accreditation status of a PA program will be listed as:

a) Continuing accreditation

A program with a continuing accreditation status is an established program in compliance with the standards of accreditation.

b) Provisional accreditation

A provisional accreditation status is granted for a limited and defined period of time to a new program that has demonstrated its preparedness to initiate a program in accordance with the standards.

c) Probationary accreditation

This is a temporary status for programs that do not meet the standards and when an acceptable educational experience for its students is threatened.

d) Developing-not accredited

Programs that are working toward accreditation, but have not yet passed the ARC-PA accreditation review. There is no guarantee that the program will be accredited.

You can find a current list of the accreditation status of every program on the Physician Assistant Education Association (PAEA) website at: *directory.paeaonline.org/programs/1019*.

2. What is the program's first-time pass/fail rate on the Physician Assistant National Certification Examination (PANCE)?

In order to become a certified physician assistant (PA-C) after you graduate from PA school, you must pass the PANCE. If you do not pass the PANCE, you cannot work as a PA; it's that simple.

So, when you are looking at programs to apply to, I strongly recommend that you consider the programs first-time pass/fail rate on the boards. The average 5-year, first-time pass/fail rates nationally are currently at 94% for all programs.

However, as you will see in Appendix 3, PA programs' first-time pass/fail rates currently range from 69% to 100%. Which program would you prefer to attend? A PANCE rate of 69% means that 3 out of 10 students who've attended that program have failed the PANCE (first-time). After accreditation status, I would consider high

PANCE rates as my second criteria. What a shame it would be to invest 2 years of your time in a program, and possibly over one hundred thousand dollars for tuition, and not be able to pass your boards and become a PA-C.

A word of caution, make sure you look at the *first-time* PANCE rates, and not the overall PANCE rates. The National Commission on Certification of Physician Assistants (NCCPA) publishes each program's PANCE rates which can be found on the program's website. The PANCE rates are typically listed over the past 5 years.

3. When did the program begin: longevity of the program?

You may be asking yourself, why is the longevity of the program so important? Won't I have a better chance of getting into a new program?

Let's consider the first question: why is longevity so important? Longevity of the program is important for a couple of reasons:

- *Track record*: A well-established program typically has (but not always) a winning formula that works to educate students and prepare them to pass the PANCE.

*Established clinical rotation sites*: It could take several years for a program to rule in, or rule out, clinical rotation sites that provide the best opportunities for their PA students to learn and have a chance to participate in the care of patients. For example, if you are on a team with interns, residents, and PA students on a surgical rotation, you may be "low man" on the totem pole when it comes to "scrubbing in" on a surgical procedure in the operating room. Some surgeons may feel an obligation to train the interns and resident first, and delegate you to the role of an observer.

Instead of being the "first-assistant" on a procedure, you may be the "third-assistant," whose job it is to hold retractors for the entire case. You may not be able to see the surgical field. You will not be able to see the anatomy, and you may not be able to practice your suturing skills.

It takes a few years for a program to weed out these rotations based on the based on the student's feedback about that particular rotation.

I found that clinical rotations play a significant role in how well you do on the PANCE, also. In your didactic training you are typically memorizing material, whereas in the clinical rotations you may remember answers to a PANCE question because you took care of a patient who had the diagnosis discussed in the question. For instance, you may be asked about the medication to treat HIV, and you will remember that medication because in your internal medicine rotation you took care of a patient with HIV and had to review her medication list every day.

4. *Is the program affiliated with a medical school?* Programs affiliated with medical schools typically have a lot more resources available to them than free-standing programs. In many cases you will take classes in conjunction with the medical students. Since a medical school is affiliated with a hospital, or hospitals, you will also have access to the medical school library and many other amenities not afforded to a free-standing program. Additionally, medical schools almost always have cadaver labs, allowing you to learn anatomy on an actual human body, versus plastic models.

5. *Does the program have a cadaver lab?* As mentioned above, learning anatomy on a cadaver is much more interesting than learning anatomy from slides or plastic models. I believe learning anatomy on a cadaver will actually make you a better clinician. You will actually see the sciatic nerve, and never forget how big it is and where it is located in the body. You will appreciate why it's important to educate your patients with sciatica to avoid placing their wallet in back pockets because of the pressure it exerts on this huge nerve. You will have the opportunity to see and touch the great vessels of the heart, heart valves, and its four chambers to gain a better understanding of how this miraculous pump works to feed blood to the body.

I will never forget the location of the *brachial plexus*, a huge bundle of nerves that run under the armpit, how it looks, and why it is so important for patients using crutches to press them on the upper side of the chest versus under the armpits, because they could damage the brachial plexus. I might not have appreciated that visual on a plastic model or a slide.

Dissecting a human cadaver is an amazing experience and a great teaching tool.

6. *Where is the program located?* If financial or family circumstances limit your ability to travel, you will probably want to apply to programs within your geographical area. I think most PA programs will

understand your circumstances, but just realize you may have to rule out-of-state programs that may be a better fit for your background, and your preferences in a program.

7. *Is it a master's program?* In the past two decades practicing as a PA, I can honestly say that I've never observed a job applicant get accepted or rejected on the basis of having a master's degree versus a bachelor's degree. There are so many job opportunities available that the only letters you need after your name are PA-C.

There are a couple of exceptions to this rule; if you want to teach at a PA program or if you want to do research, you will need a master's degree to do both.

Having said that, I certainly believe that after completing a rigorous PA program, we all probably meet or exceed the requirements for a master's degree. In fact, the trend has changed from the majority of PA programs offering bachelor's degrees, to the majority of PA programs now offering master's degrees.

In summary, I don't think it matters whether you earn a master's degree or not. I earned a graduate certificate at Yale, and not having a master's degree has never affected my clinical skills or job prospects.

8. *Who teaches the classes in the didactic phase of the program?* Many of you may not have thought about this question, or really don't see how it matters. If a program's first-time PANCE rates are 96%, who cares? I do think, however, that you should be familiar with who will provide your didactic training and what the differences may be among the various choices of educators. Here is a nonjudgmental list of options:

a) *Fellows*: A "fellow" is a physician who's completed her residency and is now investing 2 or more years learning a specialty like cardiology, dermatology, general surgery, etc.

In my opinion, who is better to teach a class in cardiology than a cardiology fellow; someone who is highly motivated and up-to-date on the most current information in the field. Additionally, since fellows are literally at the beginning of their specialized training, they are highly motivated individuals, passionate about their specialty, and less likely to suffer from "burn out."

b) *Physicians*: Many programs have local physicians who work in the community, or an affiliated medical school, lecture students in their specialty area. The benefit of having physicians teach classes in the didactic phase is that the student will benefit from that physician's many years of clinical experience.

c) *Researchers*: Researchers are probably better able to teach physiology rather than clinical medicine. These are the guys that are going to present elaborate charts and graphs and discuss the results of various clinical trials related to their field. These will be very intellectual presentations and they may keep you up late at night trying to digest the information in the lecture.

d) *Physician Assistants*: Many programs utilize physician assistants from the program or the community to teach classes. One obvious benefit of having PAs teach is the fact that they can relate better to your situation. One negative is the fact that these PAs might not have experience in the specialty course they are teaching.

9. *How much is the tuition?* In other words, consider how much debt you will be in after you graduate. Tuition varies significantly for each program, and I would certainly evaluate the "pros" and "cons" for each program you apply to or decide to attend.

10. *How much is housing, parking, and the average cost of living in the community?* These costs can add up and should be considered along with tuition expenses.

So if you're asked the question during your interview, "Why have you chosen our program?" you now have a wealth of information to draw upon when providing your answer.

## ARE YOU A GOOD FIT?

Another very important question you should ask yourself when selecting PA programs is: "Am I a good fit for this program?" What do I mean by this? As you'll see in the interview chapters, PA programs already know the qualities they're looking for in applicants they accept to their program. Your job is to find out what these qualities are, and demonstrate that you have what they're looking for. For instance, if a program's website states that they prefer to select in-state applicants and you're not from that state, your odds might not be as favorable as someone who *is* from that state. You wouldn't, necessarily, be a good fit for that program.

Additionally, if a program's mission is heavily tied into community service, and you haven't done any community service in the past, you might not be the best fit for that program. This is why it is so important to do your homework before you apply to a program. It's best to be able to *demonstrate* that you have the qualities the program is looking for. If the program values diversity, you will have a better chance for acceptance if you have a history of working with diverse populations, rather than simply saying you recognize the fact that they value diversity.

If a program has an absolute requirement of a 3.5 science GPA, and you have a 3.3 science GPA, you will not be a good fit for this program.

Don't get too worried; however, there are many programs that are more liberal when it comes to acceptance requirements.

## A NOTE ABOUT *RANKING* PA PROGRAMS

The only current media for ranking PA educational programs is *US News & World Report (US News)*. The rankings are typically updated and published every year. *US News* ranks PA programs based on a *subjective* survey of PA school faculty and administration. In my opinion, many PA school applicants, PA students, and PA faculty rely on this report as a valid indicator of a program's success. *US News & World Report* has been publishing results for the top PA programs since 1998.

In an article titled: A Novel Approach to Ranking Physician Assistant Programs (2010 Vol 21 No 4/*The Journal of Physician Assistant Education*, by James Van Rhee, MS, PA-C; Michael J. Davanzo, MMS, PA-C), a new approach to ranking PA programs was proposed based on *objective* data.

PA program directors from 126 accredited PA programs (at the time) identified indicators to include in a new ranking system for PA programs. The four criteria they agreed upon were:

1. Each program's current ARC-PA accreditation length
2. Student-to-faculty ratio
3. Percentage of faculty with doctoral degrees
4. Most recent 5-year average PANCE rates

If you take a look at Table 4.1, you can see that in 2007, the new ranking system and the *US News & World Report* ranking systems are quite different. For example, University of Wisconsin-La Crosse ranks number one in the new system, but doesn't rank in the top 20 in the *US News* system. Duke University ranks number two in the *US News & World Report* ranking system, but not in the top 20 in the new ranking system.

So what does this mean to you, the PA school applicant, when deciding to select a PA program? In my opinion, it means that you have to do your homework, and look at the four criteria listed above versus taking the *US News & World Report* data as an absolute indicator of the best PA programs.

I'm a big believer in reviewing a program's first-time PANCE rates to assess the quality of that program. If the program's PANCE rates are high (94% and above), it means they're doing an effective job of preparing students to pass the boards and ultimately become eligible to practice as a PA. I don't care how prestigious a PA program may be, or how high *US News & World Report* ranks a program, if you invest 2 or more years of your time, and possibly $100,000 or more on your education, you'll want to be sure that you will be able to pass your boards once you graduate. If you don't pass your boards, you can't work!

**Table 4.1.** Comparison of New Ranking and *US News* Ranking

| Rank | New Ranking System | Rank | *US News* Ranking 2007 |
|------|--------------------|------|------------------------|
| 1 | University of Wisconsin-La Crosse | 1 | University of Iowa |
| 2 | Oregon Health & Science | 2 | Duke University |
| 3 | University of Iowa | 3 | Emory University |
| 4 | Central Michigan University | 4 | George Washington University |
| 5 | Univ. of TX SW Medical Center | 4 | Univ. of TX SW Medical Center |
| 6 | University of Nebraska | 7 | University of Utah |
| 7 | Rutgers (UMDNJ) | 8 | University of Washington |
| 8 | University of Oklahoma—OKC | 9 | University of Colorado |
| 9 | Quinnipiac University | 9 | Baylor College of Medicine |
| 9 | Emory University | 11 | Oregon Health & Science |

**Table 4.1.** Comparison of New Ranking and *US News* Ranking *(Continued)*

| Rank | New Ranking System | Rank | *US News* Ranking 2007 |
|------|-------------------|------|------------------------|
| 11 | Desales University | 11 | Interservice PA Program |
| 12 | Duquesne University | 11 | SUNY-Stony Brook University |
| 12 | Yale University | 14 | Univ. of TX Medical Branch Galveston |
| 14 | Baylor College of Medicine | 14 | University of Nebraska |
| 14 | Augsburg College | 14 | Quinnipiac University |
| 16 | Univ. of TX Medical Branch Galveston | 17 | Rosalind Franklin University |
| 17 | SUNY-Stony Brook University | 17 | Rutgers (UMDNJ) |
| 18 | Northeastern University | 17 | Northeastern University |
| 19 | Saint Francis University (PA) | 17 | Saint Louis University |
| 20 | Wayne State University | 21 | Univ. TX Health Center San Antonio |
| 20 | Philadelphia University | 21 | Saint Francis University (PA) |

In Table 4.2, I provide you with a list of PANCE rates of the programs ranked in the top 20 for both ranking systems. Notice that the University of Wisconsin-La Crosse has 100% five-year PANCE rate and is ranked as the number one program in the new ranking system. Wisconsin-La Crosse doesn't even make the list in the *US News & World* Report ranking system, but the University of Washington with an 86% five-year PANCE rate is number seven on the *US News* list.

There are currently 19 PA programs in the country with 100% first-time pass/fail rates on the PANCE, yet only three of those programs made the *US News* top 20 list.

**Table 4.2.** Comparison of the 5-Year, First-Time Pass/Fail Rates of PA Programs in Both Ranking Systems

| New Ranking System (2016) | 5-Year PANCE Rate (%) | US News Ranking (2007) | Rank (%) |
|---|---|---|---|
| Univ. of Wisconsin-La Crosse | 100 | University of Iowa | 100 |
| Oregon Health & Science | 98 | Duke University | 96 |
| University of Iowa | 100 | Emory University | 95 |
| Central Michigan University | 96 | George Washington University | 94 |
| Univ. TX SW Medical Center | 100 | Univ. TX SW Medical Center | 100 |
| University of Nebraska | 98 | University of Utah | 93 |
| Rutgers (UMDNJ) | 97 | University of Washington | 86 |
| University of Oklahoma—OKC | 97 | University of Colorado | 98 |
| Quinnipiac University | 98 | Baylor College of Medicine | 97 |
| Emory University | 95 | Oregon Health & Science | 98 |
| Desales University | 100 | Interservice PA Program | 97 |
| Duquesne University | 92 | SUNY-Stony Brook University | 97 |
| Yale University | 98 | Univ. of TX Medical Branch-Galveston | 98 |

**Table 4.2.** Comparison of the 5-Year, First-Time Pass/Fail Rates of PA Programs in Both Ranking Systems (*Continued*)

| New Ranking System (2016) | 5-Year PANCE Rate (%) | US News Ranking (2007) | Rank (%) |
|---|---|---|---|
| Baylor College of Medicine | 97 | University of Nebraska | 98 |
| Augsburg College | 99 | Quinnipiac University | 98 |
| Univ. of TX Medical Branch-Galveston | 98 | Rosalind Franklin University | 95 |
| SUNY-Stony Brook University | 97 | Rutgers (UMDNJ) | 97 |
| Northeastern | 97 | Northeastern | 97 |
| Saint Francis University-Pennsylvania | 96 | Saint Louis University | 99 |
| Wayne State University | 96 | Univ. of TX Health Center-San Antonio | 95 |
| Philadelphia University | 94 | Saint Francis University-Pennsylvania | 96 |

# FINAL THOUGHTS ON SELECTING A PA PROGRAM

I would be remiss if I did not mention this final thought that is so important to consider when selecting a PA program. I will cover this information in greater detail in Chapter 7, but I cannot stress this concept enough. When selecting a PA program, you will definitely need to do your homework and select programs that are a good *fit* for your qualifications. As you will learn in Chapter 7, *It's not about you, it's about them!* Do you have the qualities the PA program is looking for?

PA programs already know what qualities they're looking for in candidates *before* they review your application and before you interview. It is your job to show them that you possess these qualities and that you can *demonstrate* these qualities in your essay and at the interview.

So when you begin researching programs, it is imperative that you understand what qualities each program is looking for in the perfect applicant. For instance, if you want to apply to a program that values those candidates who've worked in "underserved areas," and you have never done so, you won't satisfy their needs as compared to an applicant who's worked in soup kitchens, or has gone on missions to impoverished countries. I'm not saying you won't have a chance of getting accepted, but you won't be as strong an applicant as those who have done so.

Let's say you want to apply to Duke's PA program. If you do your homework, you will see that Duke's website, *What We Look for in an Applicant*, lists the following, specific, qualities they are seeking:

- Cultural diversity
- Applicants who are underrepresented in the PA profession
- A heart for service
- Volunteerism
- Military service
- North Carolina residents from geographically underserved areas such as Area Health Education Centers (AHEC)
- Years of experience in the health care field

These qualities are in addition to the rigorous academic, patient contact hours, and GRE scores they require.

I will cover this area in greater detail in the interview chapters, but remember that it is your job to do your research on each program you will be applying to and find out what qualities they value most. Ask yourself, "Can I *demonstrate* these qualities?" If not, you may want to look for program's where you will be a better fit or choose to get more experience in these areas before you apply.

Okay, now that you've selected your top choice programs, let's discuss the CASPA application process in this next chapter.

# CHAPTER 5

# The Application Process: The Centralized Application Service for Physician Assistants (CASPA) (caspaonline.org)

You're now ready to finally begin the application process for PA school. This is an extremely exciting time. Then you look at the CASPA application and perhaps you become intimidated by the seemingly complex process. Don't worry, you're not alone. The biggest advice I can give you is:

- apply early
- follow instructions
- pay strict attention to detail
- **read the FAQ section**

You'll find the answers to 99% of all your questions on the FAQ page. Don't be lazy; find the topic where you may have questions and read the entire section. Also, be sure to start with the *Before You Create an Application* section first.

I will also cover some of the most common CASPA FAQs at the end of this chapter.

# BACKGROUND ON THE CASPA APPLICATION

Prior to 2001, PA school applicants had to accomplish applications for each program they chose to apply to. Obviously applicants had to complete a lot of paperwork, write more than one essay, and pay a fee for every application. The cost alone certainly limited many applicants from applying to multiple programs.

In 2001, the Physician Assistant Education Association (PAEA) began using CASPA. This service allows applicants to complete a single online application, and will send the completed application to any PA program the applicant designates. In 2016 (currently), the cost for a CASPA application is 175 dollars, and 50 dollars for each additional program that utilizes CASPA.

Keep in mind that not all PA programs utilize the CASPA application at this time (about 10% ), and if you apply to one—or more—of these programs, you will have to complete a separate application and pay the appropriate fees.

You may also have to accomplish "supplemental" applications for some programs. More on this later in the chapter.

Information on the CASPA application can be found at: *portal.caspa-online.org.*

# BENEFITS OF THE CASPA APPLICATION

Since CASPA online applications became available in 2001, I've coached thousands of applicants and reviewed hundreds of CASPA applications. I've listened to the feedback from these applicants concerning the CASPA application process and why they like using this service. Here are some of the benefits you'll appreciate most:

1. The ability to apply to multiple programs using a single online application.
2. The checklist and instructions provided on the CASPA website, which simplifies the process of accomplishing the application.
3. The fact that data only has to be entered once, such as transcripts, letters of recommendation (LOR), health care experience, and demographic data.
4. The ability to access the CASPA application from any computer, update information, and save it right up until it's submitted for final verification.

## Apply Early

The CASPA application cycle runs from April every year until the following March. I strongly recommend that you start your application ASAP, even if you don't have everything you need to complete it. Many programs utilize a *rolling admissions* format; they evaluate applications as soon as they "roll" in, and they either select the applicant for an interview on the spot, or reject the applicant. Once they meet their quota for interviewees, the process is closed.

You can find a list of those programs who utilize rolling admissions on my home page (andrewrodican.com).

## Follow Instructions

Failure to follow instructions can be a fatal move on your part. Your CASPA application will not be verified until you provide all of the required information. I will provide you with some tips later in this chapter, but when all else fails, read the *Before You Create An Application* section on the CASPA website.

## Pay Strict Attention to Detail

Paying strict attention to detail is a significant quality you will need to have if you are going to be a good clinician. I know that you will be excited to get the ball rolling, and complete your application as soon as possible; however, if you rush through the process and don't pay strict attention to every detail, you will certainly regret it later.

Let me give you a personal example of the importance of paying strict attention to detail:

> After graduating from college in 1984, I made a decision to become an air force officer. I signed up at the recruiting station, and before I knew it, I was on my way to San Antonio, Texas to begin Officer Training School (OTS).
>
> OTS is an extremely intense 12-week program. In order to be a competent officer, you must exhibit many qualities required to be an effective leader. One of those qualities is the ability to pay strict attention to detail.
>
> From the first day, we were told that we would have to accomplish several measurements to show we have what it takes to become an officer. If you failed three measurements during the 12 weeks of training, you were kicked out of OTS, and you would have to join the enlisted ranks. The measurements included: physical requirements, academic requirements, and military bearing requirements.
>
> In the first week of training, we had to accomplish our first requirement: a simple multiple choice test. We were told we had only 5 minutes to complete the test. Having to answer 50 questions in 5 minutes, or 10 questions per minute, made me extremely anxious. I couldn't flunk my first measurement!
>
> The proctor handed out the exam and advised us that we could not pick up our pencils until he said "Begin," and we had to immediately drop our pencils when he said, "Stop." My heart started racing.
>
> The proctor then said, begin! I looked down at the paper and noticed a very small paragraph at the top of the page. I then glanced at the rest of the exam and read some of the seemingly simple, basic questions. Piece of cake, I thought. This almost seemed too easy.
>
> In order to complete this measurement on time, I skipped the first paragraph and began answering the questions immediately. I was a bit surprised at how easy the questions were, and I began to relax.
>
> All of a sudden I got this pit in my stomach. Something was wrong. I briefly looked up and discovered many of the other candidates had their pencils on the table and weren't answering the questions. Odd, I thought. I then refocused on the test and completed the exam well in advance of the time limit.
>
> The proctor said "Stop," and I immediately dropped my pencil. I was very happy with my performance and felt very relaxed.
>
> Then the proctor said those dreadful words that I can still hear today: If you answered *any* of these questions, you failed this measurement. My heart sank; what is he talking about. He then went on to tell us all to read that first paragraph. It clearly stated, do not pick up your pencil and do not answer any of these questions.

> I failed to pay strict attention to detail, and I flunked my first measurement.
> Two more failures and I was out. I learned my lesson and did not flunk another
> measurement during those 12 weeks.

The take home message here is to pay strict attention to detail on your
CASPA application. Read everything! Take the process step-by-step and
you'll get through it. Thousands of applicants have done it before you, and
know that you can do it too.

## Read the FAQ Section

I probably could have started and ended this entire chapter with the above
heading. Trust me, everything you need to know is on the CASPA website,
especially the FAQ section. It's laid out for you in perfect order. All you
have to do is follow directions. Enough said!

## Seven Practical Tips for Completing the CASPA Application

I'm going to provide you with seven tips to make the CASPA application
process a little easier:

1. Follow instructions. As mentioned already, take the application
   process step-by-step, follow all of the instructions, and pay strict
   attention to detail.
2. List five names of those people you plan to ask for a LOR, and be
   sure to give them a "heads up" about the format and time requirement. They really need to understand how important it is to
   accomplish their letters on time. (I will provide a complete section
   on the LOR later.)
3. Be sure to request your transcripts early and have them sent directly
   to *you*.

   The sooner you receive your transcripts, the sooner you can
   accomplish the course-work section of the application.
4. Do not exceed the 5,000-character limit on your essay. If you do, the
   remaining characters will not get entered, your essay will be cut off at
   that point, and that will show your complete lack of attention to detail.
5. Make sure that you write down the application deadlines for each
   program you are applying to and adhere to those deadlines. Otherwise, your application will not be reviewed.

6. Do your homework. Visit the websites of all the programs you've chosen, and be sure that you meet, or exceed, all of the requirements and prerequisites. Some programs won't even look at your application if you haven't met their requirements. Remember, they may get 1,000 applications and the majority of those applicants will have all of the requirements; why would they choose you, if *you* don't?

7. Apply early. Register as soon as you decide to apply to PA school, and try to get your CASPA application accomplished several weeks before each programs' application deadline, especially if they utilize rolling admissions (Appendix 4). Start acquiring the following information that you will need to accomplish the application

   a) A complete accounting of your health care experience, including number of hours accumulated (at the time of application) and dates of employment. Document dates and duties of all of your volunteer experiences as well as your shadowing experiences.

   b) Obtain a personal copy of required test scores.

   c) Collect copies of any certificates that you may have earned, including: awards, certifications (EMT, ACLS), specialized training.

   d) Obtain written transcripts ASAP.

   e) Decide whom you will choose to write your LOR. (See the next chapter for more details.)

## CASPA APPLICATION STATUS AND NOTIFICATIONS

A word of caution when it comes to notifications from CASPA: they will *not* email you if you have any incomplete data in your file. You must be proactive and frequently check the status of your application on a regular basis. The last thing you need to discover a week before a deadline is that one of your letters of reference has not been received.

To check the status of your application, open your application on the CASPA website, click on "Manage My Programs," then click on "Program Status."

The following is a list of statuses you may find:

1. IN PROGRESS
2. RECEIVED—AWAITING MATERIALS
3. MATERIALS RECEIVED—VERIFYING

4. COMPLETE DATE
5. COMPLETE DATE CURRENTLY BEING VERIFIED
6. UNDELIVERED
7. VERIFIED

## Why Is My CASPA GPA Different from the One on My Transcripts?

A lot of applicants become bewildered when they notice discrepancies between their GPA as calculated on their college transcript(s) and their GPA as calculated on the CASPA application. Why is this? If you look at the FAQ page on CASPA's website, you will see that there are four reasons for this:

1. CASPA does not recognize individual schools' forgiveness, or grade replacement policies in regards to repeated courses.
2. CASPAs numeric scale for letter grades may be different than the one used at the institutions you attended (see Table 5.1).
3. CASPA calculates all GPAs in semester hours. If you completed classes in quarter hours, CASPA will convert those grades to semester hours; 1.0 quarter hour = 0.667 semester hours.
4. CASPA breaks down your GPA by college level (freshman, sophomore, etc.). So if you attended multiple colleges and took freshman classes, they will all fall under your freshman GPA.

When calculating your GPA, CASPA utilizes:

- Quality Points (QP)
- The letter grade of each course
- The semester hours for each course
- Cumulative attempted hours for all courses

The formula is as follows:

Number of Credit Hours × Letter Grade = Quality Points
Number of Quality Points/Total Credit Hours = Calculated GPA

Please take note that a "W" counts the same as an "F" according to CASPA calculations. You can manually calculate these numbers, or you can go to my home page (andrewrodican.com) and download an excel

**Table 5.1.** CASPA Letter Grade Values

| Transcript | Letter Grade | Value |
|---|---|---|
| A+ | A | 4.0 |
| A | A | 4.0 |
| A− | A− | 3.7 |
| AB | AB | 3.5 |
| B+ | B+ | 3.3 |
| B | B | 3.0 |
| B− | B− | 2.7 |
| BC | BC | 2.5 |
| C+ | C+ | 2.3 |
| C | C | 2.0 |
| CD | CD | 1.5 |
| D+ | D+ | 1.3 |
| D | D | 1.0 |
| D− | D− | 0.7 |
| E | F | 0.0 |
| F | F | 0.0 |
| WF | F | 0.0 |

spreadsheet, put in your grades and credit hours, and your CASPA GPA will automatically be calculated for you.

# LETTERS OF RECOMMENDATION (LOR)

As part of the CASPA application process, you are required to provide at least three LOR in support of your application. Be sure to pay strict attention to detail relevant to each school's specific requirements for whom they want as referees. For example, some programs may allow you to choose from your own personal references. Others may specify that you will need letters from a PA, a physician, and a former supervisor.

When considering candidates to provide your LOR, I advise that you ask at least one PA to write it (unless otherwise specified). After all, who is better to write about the qualities you possess to become a good PA than a physician assistant? Additionally, the PA profession is made up of a tight-knit, and protective, group of health care professionals. We want to be sure that if we recommend an applicant for PA school, that person is a high-quality applicant. So, an LOR from a PA probably carries the most weight with respect to any other choices. Unfortunately, many applicants fail to realize the importance of securing an LOR from a PA. Many applicants will write about shadowing a PA in their essay, but fail to include a recommendation letter from that person in their CASPA application.

Another huge mistake some PA school applicants make when selecting individuals to write their LOR is to assume the bigger the name or status of the referrer (the "big shot"), the more weight the LOR will carry. Nothing could be further from the truth!

Let me give you an example of what I mean. Some applicants will ask a big shot to write an LOR for them. The big shot agrees, and all is well. The applicant feels confident the LOR from this person is going to boost his chances.

Then 1 week before the school's deadline, the applicant realizes his CASPA application has not been verified. He's still missing one LOR. Guess whose letter is missing? That's right, the big shot. Now what? The big shot is typically unavailable to take your phone calls, she is not responding to your emails, and because she is a big shot, you are afraid of being too pushy.

Be sure you will feel comfortable contacting your referees, if they are cutting it close to the deadline, and give them a little push to get the letter of recommendation submitted as soon as possible.

## What Should be Included in Your Letter of Recommendation?

I recommend that the writer of your LOR comment on the following areas:

- Academic performance
- Interpersonal skills
- Maturity

- Adaptability and flexibility
- Motivation for a career as a PA
- Ability to work collaboratively with others
- Strengths relative to a career as a PA

A strong LOR also includes four specific features:

1. It shows that the writer genuinely knows the individual and can comment about the applicant's qualifications.
2. It shows the writer knows enough about the applicant and can make comparative judgments about the applicant's intellectual, academic, and professional abilities in relation to others in a similar role.
3. It provides supporting details to make the statement believable.
4. It is short, yet concise and sincere.

## Who Should Write Your Letter of Recommendation?

Believe it or not, not everyone you ask to write an LOR for you is going to write a positive one. I have personally witnessed this first hand while serving on the admissions committee at Yale. Why does this happen? In my experience, many of you tend to look at the requirement of obtaining three LOR simply as a box to be checked off on the application, instead of putting thought into who would provide you with the best (positive and favorable) recommendation. Some of you will also wait until the last minute, and feel pressured to ask *anyone* to write your LOR simply to meet the requirement.

Let me provide you with some tips on how to obtain the best LOR:

1. You must know how to ask for it. I recommend you ask the potential referrer: *"Professor Jones, do you feel you can write a <u>strong and favorable</u> letter of recommendation for my candidacy to PA school?"* By asking this way, Professor Jones may feel a certain obligation to commit to writing a strong and favorable letter.

    If professor Jones feels as though he cannot commit to writing a strong and favorable letter of recommendation in support of your candidacy, he will likely refuse. This will be a blessing in disguise, as you won't be surprised to find out that professor Jones wrote an *unfavorable* letter. His refusal will provide you with an opportunity to find another referee who *will* provide a positive letter of recommendation.

2. You must know this person well and feel confident that this person knows you well enough to make specific comments on your qualities to become a competent PA student/PA.

3. You must ask the referrer early in the application process in order to ensure the letter of recommendation is submitted on time. Be sure you feel comfortable enough with each person you choose to confront them if the deadline is approaching and she hasn't submitted it to CASPA yet.

4. Make it easy for the referrer to write the letter. Provide bullet points on your qualities that the referrer can place directly into the letter. See Appendix 5 for a list of effective phrases and the five categories that should be covered in a strong letter of recommendation.

5. Write it yourself! That's right, if you want a strong and positive letter of recommendation, who is better to write it than you? You may think this is a bit forward, but it's really a common practice. Of course you must first *feel out* the person you ask to write your letter of recommendation. Get a sense of how they might react to your request. You may want to say, "*Sue, I know you are extremely busy and your time is valuable. I would certainly be willing to compose a draft letter and you could, obviously, make any changes you feel appropriate.*" Now, if you know Sue well, you should be comfortable with this proposal.

In my experience, I always feel grateful when someone volunteers to write his own LOR. Why? I am extremely busy, and I like this person and want to do an effective job with my recommendation; it will take some time to create the letter. I welcome any help. Of course if I disagree with anything in the letter, I will make the appropriate changes.

In the next chapter we are going to cover one of the most stressful components of the CASPA application; the essay.

# CHAPTER 6

# The Essay: Your Ticket to the Interview

Your PA school essay may be the most important piece of medical writing that you will ever accomplish. I have been reviewing PA school applicant essays for over 20 years now, both as an admissions committee member myself, and as a PA school applicant coach. On many occasions, the only thing standing between you and an invitation to interview is your essay.

Because the essay is so important to your candidacy, I asked the team at IvyEssays (IvyEssays.com) to write this chapter of the book. IvyEssays are admissions experts who've spent years integrating the advice of admissions counselors from the nation's top schools. They have also compiled thousands of essays from applicants who've already been accepted to these schools.

I partnered with IvyEssays several years ago and we've helped hundreds of PA school applicants. We get applicants interviews!

NOTE: Although the following material is directed at medical students, the material is equally relevant to physician assistant school students. If you like, just change the word "medical student/school" to "PA student/school," and the message will remain the same.

PA school applicants can utilize the services of IvyEssays by clicking on my website, andrewrodican.com, or by going directly to IvyEssays.com. When you submit your essay for editing, be sure to mention my name in the comments box so IvyEssays will know exactly how to edit your PA school essay.

# GENERAL TIPS FOR WRITING SUCCESSFUL ESSAYS

- Express Motivation
- Demonstrate Effective Communication Skills
- Discuss Your Soft Skills
- Be Real
- Be Personal
- Use Details
- Tell a Story
- Be Honest

During the first, quick look at your file (transcripts, science and non-science GPAs, MCAT GRE scores, application, recommendations, and personal statement,) what the admissions committee seeks is essentially the same:

"Proven ability to succeed."

"Clear intellectual ability, analytical and critical thinking skills"

"Evidence that this person has the potential to make not just a good medical student, but a good doctor"

But what they look for when they hone in on your essay is much more than this. We will discuss in detail the things that were unanimously listed as being the most important by our admissions committee.

## Express Motivation

Your application to medical school (PA school) is a testimony to your desire to ultimately become a doctor (PA). The admissions committee will look to your essay to see that you've demonstrated the obvious—but not so simple—question "why?" You must be able to explain your motivation for attending medical school (PA school).

"I look for a sustained understanding of why the candidate wants to enter medicine, how they've tested their interest, and how they've prepared for medical school (PA school)."

"Touch on your passion to pursue medicine. For many medicine is akin to a calling, and it is compelling for the evaluator to sense that they are hearing and responding to the same motivation."

You will be offered much advice in the upcoming pages, and it will be peppered with plenty of "dos" and "don'ts." In the midst of all of this, whatever you do, don't lose sight of the ultimate goal of the essay: you must convince the admissions committee that you belong at their medical (PA) school. Everything we tell you should be used as a means to this end, so step back from the details regularly to remind yourself of the big picture:

"The essay is the venue for the candidate to make the argument as to why they, among all the qualified candidates, should be admitted to medical school (PA school) and the eventual practice of medicine."

## Demonstrate Effective Communication Skills

Another obvious function of the essay is to showcase your language abilities and writing skills.

"In the essay I want a clear sense that they understand and can communicate well why they are a compelling candidate."

"Especially if they did some or all of their prerequisite coursework in another country, we will look to the essay to ensure strong English language skills."

But at this level, good writing skills are not sought—they are expected. So while a beautifully written essay isn't going to get you into medical school (PA school), a poorly written one could keep you out of it.

Beyond showcasing your writing abilities and demonstrating your motivation, what else can the essay do for you? Let's take a look at what else the committee hopes to find when they pick your essay.

## Discuss Your Soft Skills

Let the rest of your application—not the personal statement—speak for your "hard" skills and achievements (i.e., your academic excellence, your fantastic MCAT (GRE) scores, your class rank). What they seek in the essay are some specific "soft" skills such as maturity, empathy, compassion, depth, and motivation. These qualities were rated especially high in the medical community— more so than any other graduate-level program we studied (Table 6.1).

These qualities are not quantifiable, and therefore not easily demonstrated.

All of the essays we have in our database demonstrate in one way or another that the writers have the soft skills necessary to be good doctors (PAs). A few of them even come right out and say it:

"Motivation, independence, maturity, precisely those qualities my experiences in Eastern Europe instilled, will be essential to a fruitful career."

But when qualities are mentioned as directly as this, the applicant must be careful to support the claims with clear evidence as gathered from

**Table 6.1.** Qualities Rated High in the Medical Field

| 1 | 2 | 3 |
|---|---|---|
| Motivation | Diversity | Sensitivity |
| Commitment | Uniqueness | Communication skills |
| Sincerity | Interest | Humanitarian beliefs |
| Honesty | Compassion | Enthusiasm |
| Maturity | Empathy | Creativity |

their personal experience. Most often they just let their achievements speak for themselves, and the qualities that they demonstrate are inferred.

## Be Real

The list is not ordered by importance—if it was, this category would be listed first. More than any specific skill or characteristic, what our admissions panel said they seek more than anything else in the personal statement is a real, live human being:

"The members of a medical admissions committee are responsible for choosing the next generation of medical doctors (PAs). These are the people who will be healing our children, curing our parents, and literally saving lives. Put it in that perspective and the responsibility we feel is enormous. For this reason, we're going to choose to accept someone we feel we know, trust, and like."

In light of this, then, it might not surprise you that when we asked admissions officers and medical students for their #1 piece of advice regarding the essay, we received the same response almost every time. Although it was expressed in many different ways (be honest, be sincere, be unique, be personal, etc.), it all came down to the same point: "Be Yourself!"

"My #1 piece of advice is: BE YOURSELF WHEN YOU WRITE THE ESSAY...THE MEDICAL PROFESSION IS A LIFETIME COMMITMENT...LET THEM TRULY KNOW WHAT DRIVES YOU TOWARD IT!!!!!"

Unfortunately, achieving this level of communication in writing does not come naturally to everyone. But that does not mean it cannot be learned. Once you understand the basic factors that go into personable writing you will see that it is not as hard as it seems.

NOTE: Part of what can make this kind of writing seem so difficult is that it is very hard to gauge the image you are projecting through your writing. Even if you have followed every tip in this chapter, it is a good idea to have someone objective—preferably someone who doesn't already know you well—read it over when you have finished. Ask them if they got a sense of the kind of person you are, or if they were able to picture you as they were reading. How accurate is their description to the one you you're trying to present? Then ask them if the person they pictured is someone that they would choose to be treated by in a life or death situation!

## Be Personal

The only way to let the admissions committee see you as an individual is to make your essay personal. When you do this your essay will automatically be more interesting and engaging, helping it stand out from the hundreds of others the committee will be reviewing that week.

"After reading hundreds of essays in my time on the Harvard Medical School (HMS) admissions committee, I would tell people a couple of key things. First, make it personal. The most boring, dry essays are those that go on about how they love science and working with people and want to serve humanity, but give few personal details that give a sense of what the applicant is like."

"Personalize your essay as much as possible—generic essays are not only boring to read, they're a waste of time because they don't tell you anything about the applicant that helps you get to know them better."

But what does it mean to make your essay personal? It means that you drop the formalities and write about something that is truly meaningful to you. It means that you include a story or anecdote taken from your life, using lots of details and colorful imagery to give it life. And it means, above all, being completely honest.

Our database contains many examples of essays that get personal. The following example is one of them. The writer begins by recollecting her experience with anorexia and her admiration for the doctor who saved her life. But it is more than this story that makes her essay real, it is the way that she describes her experiences. She uses a real, personal tone throughout the essay, for example, when she describes herself while volunteering at an AIDS clinic.

"...I am constantly reminded about how much I have to learn. I look at a baby and notice it's cute, pudgy toes. Dr. V. plays with it while conversing with its mother, and in less than a minute has noted its responsiveness, strength, and attachment to its parent, and checked its reflexes, color, and hydration. Gingerly I search for the tympanic membrane in the ears of a cooperative child and touch an infant's warm, soft belly, willing my hands to have a measure of Dr. V.'s competence."

It is her admittance that she doesn't know everything she needs to know coupled with the picture she paints of herself noticing a baby's "cute pudgy toes" and "gingerly" searching in "the ear of a cooperative child" and touching "an infant's warm, soft belly." It is hard not to get a feel of the individual behind the who painted such a vivid portrayal using personal details.

Just as this writer did not rely on her tale of anorexia to make her essay personal, as one admissions officer put it:

"A personal epiphany, tragedy, life change, or earth shattering event is not essential to a strong essay."

This cannot be stressed enough. Personal does not have to mean heavy, or emotional, or even inspiring. It is a small minority of students who will truly have had a life-changing event to write about. Perhaps they had spent time living abroad or have experienced death or disease from close proximity. But this is the exception, not the rule.

In fact, students who rely too heavily on these weighty experiences often do themselves an injustice. They often don't think about what has really touched them or interests them because they are preoccupied with the topic that they think will impress the committee. They write about their grandfather's death because they think that only death (or the emotional equivalent) is significant enough to make them seem deep and mature. But what often happens is they rely on the experience itself to speak for them and never explain what it meant to them or give a solid example of how it changed them. In other words, they don't make it personal.

## Use Details

To make your essay personal, learn from the example above and use details. Show, don't tell, who you are by backing your claims with real past experiences.

"Essays only help if they are unique and enable the interviewer to get a sense of who the person is based on examples and scenarios and ideas, rather than lists of what they've done. The readers want to find out WHO THIS PERSON IS; not what they've done, although the two are obviously interrelated."

The key words from the quote are: "examples," scenarios," and "ideas." Using details means getting specific. Each and every point that you make needs to be backed up by specific instances taken from your experience. It is these details that make your story special, unique, and interesting.

Look at the detail used in the following example. The writer takes care to describe herself gently rocking her first patient, "taking care not to disturb the jumbled array of tubes that overwhelmed his tiny body," and that she has "worked with everything from papier mache to popsicle sticks" and that the children in her ward talk about "Nintendo or the latest Disney movie." This is the difference between a personal, interesting treatment of a story, and a yawn-inducing account that could be attributed to any of a thousand applicants.

## Tell a Story

"Tell a story, it always makes for more interesting reading and it usually conveys something more personal than blanket statements like 'I want to help people'."

Incorporating a story into your essay can be a great way to make it interesting and enjoyable. The safest and most common method of integrating a story into an essay is to tell the story first, then step back into the role of narrator and explain why it was presented and what lessons were learned. The reason this method works is that it forces you to begin with the action, which is a surefire way to get the reader's attention and keep them reading.

Many of the essay examples in our database (Appendix 6) make effective use of storytelling. One begins with a storm at sea, one with a tale of stage fright before a theater performance, and one with a newspaper clipping about the writer as a child. Another writer takes an even more creative approach to the story method by incorporating the story of a prehistoric woman whose bones he has analyzed throughout the entire essay. What all these writers understood is that a story is best used to draw the reader in. It should always relate back to the motivation to attend medical (PA) school or the ability to succeed once admitted.

## Be Honest

This last tip comes with no caveats, and should be upheld without exception. Nothing could be more simple, more straightforward, or more crucial than this: be honest, forthright, and sincere.

Admissions officers have zero tolerance for hype. If you try to be something that you're not, it will be transparent to the committee. You will come off as immature at best and as unethical at worst. "If you say that one of your favorite hobbies is playing chess, then you better have a favorite opening move...your interviewer may be an expert player and want to swap techniques!"

"I served on the Harvard Med admissions committee, and can say that it is so important to be honest. The students will be asked many times about the personal statement when interviewing, and it's painfully obvious when they exaggerate or are overly dramatic when recounting their experiences."

When you are honest about your motivation and goals, you will come across as more personable and real. One essayist, for example, begins:

"When I entered Dartmouth College in 1987, I was amazed by the large number of students already labeled as 'pre-meds.' I wondered how those students were able to decide with such certainty that they wanted to study medicine, and I imagined that they all must have known from a very early age that they would one day be great doctors. I had no such inklings, and if asked as a child what I wanted to be when I grew up, I would have said that I wanted to be an Olympic skier or soccer player."

Because of the plethora of essays that begin: "I've wanted to be a doctor for as long as I can remember..." this writer's honesty must have been refreshing and memorable.

## SELECTING AN ESSAY TOPIC

- Getting Started
- Assessing Yourself
- Identifying Your Themes
- Developing a Strategy
- Avoiding Pitfalls

### Getting Started

To get the most benefit out of this section, put your anxieties aside. Don't think about what the admissions committee wants, don't worry about grammar or style, and especially don't worry about what anyone would think. Worries like these hamper spontaneity and creativity. Focus instead on writing quickly and recording every thought you have the instant you have it. You will know that you are performing these exercises correctly if you are relaxing and having fun.

## Stream of Consciousness

Take 20 minutes to answer each of the questions: Who are you? and What do you want? Start with whatever comes to mind first, and without pausing for the entire time. Don't limit yourself to any one area of your life such as your career. Just let yourself go, be honest, and have fun. You might be surprised by what kind of results can come from this type of free association.

## Morning Pages

If you have the discipline to practice this technique for a week, you may end up doing it for the rest of your life. Keep a paper and a pen at your bedside. Set your alarm clock 20 minutes early, and when you are still in bed and groggy with sleep, start writing. Write about anything that comes to mind, as fast as you can, and do not stop until you have filled a page or two.

## Journal Writing

Keep a journal for a few weeks, especially if you are stuck and your brainstorming seems to be going nowhere. Record not what you do each day but your responses and thoughts about each day's experiences.

## Top Tens

Write down your top 10 favorites in the following areas: movies, books, songs, musicians, sports, paintings, historical areas, and famous people. Step back and look at the lists objectively. What do they say about you? Which favorites are you most passionate about? How have these favorites affected your outlook, opinions, or direction?

## Free-Flow Writing

Choose a word from your questions such as "influence," strengths," "career," "diversity," or "goals" and brainstorm around it. Set a timer for

10 minutes and write without stopping. Write down everything that you can think of that relates to the topic, including any single words that come to mind.

## Assessing Yourself

Hopefully the exercises in the last section successfully stirred your thoughts and animated your pen. If so, then it is time to impose more focus on your brainstorming. These next exercises help you do just that. They concentrate on finding the specific points and details that can be used to answer each of your questions. But as you work on them be sure to retain the open mind and creative attitude with which you approached the last exercises.

First, make a list of all the questions you have to answer for each school, leaving plenty of space next to each. Work on the following exercises proactively, keeping these questions in mind as you write. When you have uncovered a point or example that could potentially be used in response to one of them, make a note of it next to the question and then go right back to the brainstorming. If you can apply one situation or experience to multiple questions, do so. Don't censor yourself. At this stage of the writing process, more is better—you can worry about honing and culling later. The objective now is to accumulate multiple items for each question.

### The Chronological Method

Start from childhood and record any and all special or pivotal experiences that you remember. Go from grade to grade, and job to job, noting any significant lessons learned, achievements reached, painful moments endured, or obstacles overcome. Also, include your feelings about those occurrences as you remember them. If you are a visual person, it might help to draw a timeline. Do not leave out any significant event.

Because so many questions ask about your past, this exercise can help you uncover material that will likely be used in several places. A few schools will ask you directly about your childhood and have you highlight a memory from your youth. Don't automatically discount memories that you think will seem trite or silly. A childhood memory could be used, for example, to demonstrate a long-standing passion or to emphasize how an aspect of your character is so ingrained that it has been with you since youth.

## *Assess Your Accomplishments*

Write down anything you are proud of doing, no matter how small or insignificant it might seem. Do not limit your achievements to your career. If you have overcome a difficult personal obstacle, be sure to list this too. If something is important to you, it speaks volumes about who you are and what makes you tick. Some accomplishments will be obvious, such as any achievement that received public acknowledgment. Others are less so, and many time the defining moments of our lives are those we are inclined to dismiss.

# List Your Skills

Do a similar assessment of your skills that you did for your accomplishments. Begin by looking at the accomplishments you listed for the last exercise and listing the skills that these accomplishments demonstrate. When you have a list of words start brainstorming on specific scenarios that demonstrate these skills. Pretend that you are defending these skills in front of a panel of judges. Stop only when you have proven each point to the best of your ability. Some of your skills will be obvious, such as artistic, musical, or athletic abilities. Others will be more subtle (but just as important!).

## *Analyze Personality Traits*

Take advantage of the often fuzzy distinction between skills and personality traits, and if you are having trouble listing and defending your skills, shift the focus to your qualities and characteristics instead.

Make a few columns on a sheet of paper. In the first one, list some adjectives you would use to describe yourself. In the next one, list the words your best friend would use. Use the other columns for other types of people—perhaps one for your favorite teacher and another for family members or classmates.

When you are done, see which words come up the most often. Then group them together and list the different situations in which you have exhibited these characteristics. How effectively can you illustrate or prove that you possess these qualities? Proving your points is important.

## *Note Major Influences*

You can refer back to your "Top Ten" lists for help getting started with this exercise. Did a particular book or quote make you rethink your life? Was there a particular person who shaped your values and views?

Relationships can be good material for an essay, particularly one that challenged you to look at people in a different way. Perhaps you had a wise and generous mentor from whom you learned a great deal. Have you had an experience that changed how you see the world, or defines who you are? What details of your life, special achievements, and pivotal events have helped shape you and influenced your goals?

## Identify Your Goals

The first step of this exercise is to let loose and write down anything that comes to mind in response to the following questions: What are your wildest dreams? What did you want to be when you were a kid? If you could do or be anything right now, regardless of skill, money, or other restrictions, what would it be? Think as broadly as you wish, and do not limit yourself to career goals. Will you have kids? What kind of house will you live in and what kinds of friends will you have? What would you do if you were so rich that you didn't have to work?

# Identifying Your Themes

Part of what makes the personal statement so difficult is that you need to do so much in one essay. Unlike the college application essay, where your motivation is unquestioned and your goals can remain undefined, and unlike other graduate programs where you are expected to write multiple essays in response to specific questions, writing a personal statement requires that you incorporate multiple themes in one composition. Needless to say, this can be tricky.

There are three basic themes that need to be incorporated into your essay. The first addresses the question "Why do you want to be a doctor (PA)? The second addresses "Why are you unique, different, or exceptional?" and the third "Why are you qualified?" and/or "What experience have you had?"

There are several different ways to approach each one of these themes. The more common of these approaches are outlined below with tips and advice for how to best handle each approach.

### Theme 1: Why I want to be a Doctor (PA)

Many people look back to cite the moment of their initial inspiration. Some people have wanted to be a doctor (PA) for so long they don't even know what originally inspired them. To incorporate this theme, look back to the material you gathered in the last section, specifically in response to

"The Chronological Method," "Note Major Influences," and Identify Your Goals." Ask yourself these questions: How old was I when I first wanted to be a doctor (PA)? Was there a defining moment? Was there ever any ambivalence? Was I inspired by a specific person? What kind of doctor (PA) do I want to be and how does that tie into my motivation?

Here are a few of the common ways that students incorporate this theme:

"I've always wanted to be a doctor (PA).

AKA: "I've wanted to be a doctor (PA) since I was..." and "Everyone has always said I'd be a good doctor (PA)."

This is perhaps the most common approach of all. The secret to doing it well is to show, not just tell, why you want to be a doctor (PA). You can't just say it and expect it to stand on its own.

"The 'I've always wanted to be a doctor (PA) essay has been done to death. I think such candidates need to be careful that their decision was not only a preadolescent one and has been tested over the years and approached in a mature manner."

Supply believable details from your life to make your desire real to the reader. One secret to avoiding the "here we go again" reaction is to be particularly careful with your first line. Starting with "I've wanted to be a doctor (PA) since..." makes them cringe. It's an easy line to fall back on, but admissions officers have read this sentence more times than they care to count—don't add to the statistic.

"My Parents are Doctors (PAs)..."

This approach to the "Why I want to be a doctor (PA)" theme is dangerous for a different reason.

"It's a prejudice of mine, but the legacy essay, the one that reads 'my Dad and my grandpa and my great-grandpa were all doctors (PAs) so I should be too' makes me suspect immaturity. I envision a young person who can't think for themselves or make up their own minds."

This is not the opinion of every officer, though. The point isn't to avoid admitting that your parent is an MD (PA), it is to avoid depending on that as the sole reason for you wanting to go to medical (PA) school. If a parent truly was your inspiration, then explain why you were inspired. One essay in our database takes a unique approach—he tells of how he initially revolted about becoming a doctor because of family pressure to do so. His story of how he eventually came around to the decision on his own terms makes for an interesting and convincing read.

"My Doctor Changed My Life!"

AKA: "Being a patient made me want to become a doctor."

Some people are motivated to become doctors because they have had a personal experience of illness or disability.

"I had a student who grew up with a chronic illness. She spent much time with physicians and other health care providers throughout her young life. In her essay she wrote about this continuing experience and how the medical professionals treated her. She wrote of her admiration of them as well as her understanding that they couldn't yet cure her. Her essay literally jumped off the page as being unique to her and a compelling understanding of and testament to her desire to join the people who had been so important to her life."

If your personal experience with the medical industry sincerely is your motivation for attending medical (PA) school, then do write about it. The problem is that many students fall back on this topic even when it doesn't hold particularly true for them. We can't stress enough that you do not have to have a life-defining ability or a dramatic experience to have an exciting statement. Admissions committees receive piles of accident- and illness-related essays and the ones that seem insincere stick out like sore thumbs (pun intended!) and do not reflect well on you as a candidate.

"My orthodontist changed my life!" "My dentist gave me a smile back!" These types of themes are certainly valid, but go beyond that to what particular aspect of the profession intrigues you. Do you understand how many years of study your orthodontist had to endure to reach his level of practice? Have you observed your dentist for any significant amount of time? Do you know that the profession now is much different than it was when he was starting out? Have you given any thought to the danger of infectious diseases to all health care professionals? Present a well-organized, complete essay.

One of the essayists in our database begins with a line that is often overused, and makes it the subject of the first paragraph. What makes it work is that he moves briskly in the next paragraph to demonstrate that he balanced his initial inspiration with real hospital experience. This taught him that being a doctor is more about hard work and commitment than about the good feeling of being cured or curing.

Another of our essayists describes her experience with illness in vivid language to capture the reader's interest:

"The morning of New Year's Day, 1978, was bright and sunny. Refreshed from a good night's sleep, I lifted the blankets, rose to my feet, and collapsed, unable to walk."

She does not dwell on the experience, though, and like the others provides plenty of further evidence of her sincere motivation.

Another demonstrates the most personal patient experience of them all: she suffered from anorexia and "slowly came to realize that my pediatrician had saved my life—despite my valiant efforts to the contrary." Her story works because she tells her story objectively and with no intention to manipulate the reader's emotions.

"My Mom Had Cancer"

This theme is really just a variation of "I was a patient myself" and the same advice applies: If a loved one's battle with illness, trauma, or a disability is truly what inspired your wish to become a doctor (PA), then by all means mention it. But don't dwell on it, don't over-dramatize, and don't let it stand as your sole motivation—show that you've done your research and you understand the life of a doctor (PA) and choose it for a variety of reasons.

Two of our essayists mention their sister's struggles very briefly (one with cancer and one mentally challenged) but neither spends more than a couple of sentences on the subject. Another begins with the story of a teacher suffering from AIDS. What validates this focus is the writer's subsequent involvement as a volunteer at an HIV clinic—without this evidence to prove her sincerity, the poignancy of the situation would have been doubted and the essay considerably weakened.

"I Want to Help People"

It is common and natural to cite a desire to help people. Many of the essayists in our database do just this. Perhaps the most poignant and convincing of the group is the applicant who writes of his involvement with three boys as part of a volunteer program. It is easy to see how such a person would make a kind, caring, and involved physician (physician assistant). Another essayist compares being a doctor to being a minister—it rings sincere when we discover that he himself is an elder in his church.

## The Medical Dichotomy

One of the major draws of the medical field is the dualistic nature combining hard-core science with the softer side of helping people. This is described by people in many ways: some describe it as a dichotomy of science to art. To others, it's intellectualism to humanism, theory to application, research to creativity, or qualitative to social skills. No matter how you choose to phrase it, if you mention the dichotomy, then be sure to touch on your qualifications and experience in both areas.

## Theme 2: Why am I an Exceptional Person?

This theme is often tied in closely with "why I am a qualified person." Be very clear on the difference, though the latter focuses specifically on your experience (medical or otherwise) that qualifies you to be a better medical (PA) student, while this one focuses strictly on you as a person. Committees are always on the lookout for well-rounded candidates. They want to see that you are interesting, involved, and tied to the community around you.

To help you think how to support this theme, look at the answers to the exercises from the last chapter and ask yourself: What makes me different? Do I have any special talents or abilities that might make me more interesting? How will my skills and personality traits add diversity to the class? What makes me stand out from the crowd? How will this help me to be a better doctor (PA) and student?

If you are creative, you'll be able to take whatever makes you different—even a flaw—and turn it to your advantage.

"One student wrote about her experience as a childhood klutz and how her many accidents kept her continually in medical care. The care she received was the impetus to her desire to be a doctor (PA) and made her essay entertaining, sincere, and eminently credible."

Note that the candidate in this example tied her experience into her desire to become a doctor. It is imperative that this is done with practically every point you make in your essay.


## The Talented Among Us

If you are one of a lucky few who have an outstanding talent or ability, now is no time to hide it. Whether you are a star athlete, an opera singer, or a violin virtuoso, by all means make it a focus of your essay.

"These people can be some of the strongest of candidates. Assuming, always, that they've excelled in the required preparatory coursework, the other strengths can take them over the top. Athletes, musicians, etc. can make the compelling case of excellence, achievement, discipline, mastering a subject/talent, and leveraging their abilities. Medical schools are full of these types—they thrive by bringing high achievers who possess intellectual ability into their realm."

If you do plan to focus on a strength outside the field of medicine, your challenge becomes one of how to tie the experience of that ability into your motivation for becoming a doctor.

One of our essayists begins with a description of an African drumming performance during a Catholic mass, and then ties back to the musical theme nicely in the last line. Music was a profound interest in the life of another writer, and she rightly devotes her theme to the healing power of music and her study of musical therapy.

Another essayist draws a compelling portrait of an avid skier and swimmer and effectively ties her interest in sports to medicine through her experience as a life guard and a member of the emergency medical ski team.

## Students of Diversity

If you are diverse in any sense of the word: if you are an older applicant, a minority, a foreign applicant, or disabled, use it to your advantage by showing what your unique background will bring to the school and to the practice of medicine. Some admissions officers, however, warn against using minority status as a qualification instead of quality. If you fall into this trap, your diversity will work against you.

Building a bridge between the two. "If you are a 'student of diversity' then of course, use it. But don't harp on it for its own sake or think that being diverse by itself is enough to get you in—that will only make us feel manipulated and it will show that you didn't know how to take advantage of a good opportunity."

So just be sure you tie it in with either your motivation or your argument for why it makes you a better candidate, you will be standing on safe ground.

## Late Comers and Career Switchers

Luckily for all of us, you needn't be a minority, a foreign applicant, disabled, or an athlete or musician to be considered diverse. There are, for example, those who have had experience in or prepared themselves for totally different fields. One of our essays was written by a management consultant who was looking to switch careers. Another begins by telling how miserable he was as a branch manager for a marketing corporation. Another is written by a woman who had always planned to go into Public Health, and yet another originally wanted to be a veterinarian. All of them give succinct reasons for wanting to shift into medicine and show evidence of sincere and intensive preparation for their new chosen field.

## English Majors and Theater People

Not everyone who is accepted to medical school has a hard-core science background. One essayist wanted to be a writer originally and writes persuasively on the similarities between analyzing literature and analyzing medical research. He takes this one step further when discussing the creative versus the analytical approach to medicine and his lofty ambition of building a bridge between the two. One essay opens with the author's involvement in a play, and openly admits that she was initially turned off by science and math. Another was a Classics major and another admits that she "turned away from science during my undergraduate years."

The secret of all these essays is that they know how to turn their potential weaknesses into strengths. They point out that communication is an integral part of being a doctor, and discuss the advantages of their well-rounded backgrounds. They are also very careful to demonstrate their motivation and qualifications in detail and with solid evidence to offset worries that their non-science backgrounds have given them an unrealistic view of a doctor's life or that their ability to cope with the science courses at medical school will be compromised.

## Can I Be too Well-Rounded?

Some people have talents, abilities, or experience in so many different areas that they risk coming across as unfocused or undedicated. When handled deftly, though, your many sides can be brought together, and what could have hurt you ends up setting you apart instead. One of our essayists does a terrific job of this. She was an Art History major, active in varsity sports, health education, and traveling. She'd been an Au Pair in Iceland and an exchange student and intern in France. She manages to present all of this in a short, pointed essay by using the concept of "connections" as her theme. She relates systems of connections both to the human body as well as to her own diverse activities, emphasizing how they all come together to form a coherent and unique whole.

## Taking Advantage of International Experience

Many applicants have international experience. So while it may not set you apart in a totally unique way, it is always worthwhile to demonstrate your cross-cultural experience and sensitivity. Many in our database have written descriptions of their foreign experience ranging from volunteering in Africa, Brazil, and Honduras to au pairing in Iceland to opera singing in Paris. One essay is especially strong in the area of international experience. This exceptional man worked as a farmhand in Hungary and an orderly in the Former Soviet Union, financed by the first hospital in Estonia, and organized a mission to deliver medical supplies to refugees in Bosnia.

Notice again, though, that all these essayists went beyond simply writing about their experiences to relating them either to their motivation or qualifications. Don't expect the committee to make these leaps for you—you need to put it in your own words and make the connection clear.

## Religion

Some admissions counselors advise avoiding mention of religion altogether. Others say that it can be used to an applicant's advantage by setting them apart and by stressing values and commitment. This is a somewhat touchy subject area and is best left to the individual choice. A few of our essayists mention religion to varying degrees. One was a missionary for the Church of Latter-day Saints for 2 years and another is an elder of the same. The last merely mentions Bible-study in passing, so-to-speak, but it still sheds light on what is probably an important part of her life.

## Theme 3: Why I Am a Qualified Person?

The last major theme deals with your experience and qualifications both for attending medical (PA) school and for becoming a good doctor (PA). Having direct hospital or research experience is always the best evidence you can give. If you haven't, then consider what other experience you have that is related. Have you been a volunteer? Have you tutored English as a second language? Were you a teaching assistant? The rule to follow here is: if you have done it, use it.

## Hospital/Clinical Experience

Direct experience with patients is probably the best kind to have in your essay. What is important to notice in the essays in our database is that any kind or amount of experience was mentioned, no matter how insignificant it might appear. Some essayists even cite experience they gained in high school. Many are volunteers, some as HIV counselors, some in emergency rooms, some as lab assistants, and some simply escorted patients to their correct rooms.

## Research Experience

A word of caution: don't focus solely on your research topic—your essay will become impersonal at best and downright dull at worst. Watch out for overuse of what non-science types refer to as "medical garble." If it's necessary for the description of your project then of course, you have no choice. But throwing medical terms around just because you can won't impress anyone. Good writers can delve into the use of scientific and medical terms, but they also spend plenty of time away from them as well, sounding like real human beings.

### Unusual Medical Experience

Even if you haven't put in X number of hours a week at a clinic or spent a term on a research project, you might still have medical experience that counts, like the time you cared for your sick grandmother or the day you saved the man at the next table from choking in a restaurant. It doesn't even matter if you were unsuccessful (maybe, despite your valiant efforts, the man at the next table didn't survive) if it was meaningful to you then it was relevant. In fact, three essays in our database relay tales of failing to save a life. One, on the other hand, relays a fascinating success story: the writer was forced to become a doctor by default to a village in Honduras for a summer, even though she had no formal training, no experience, and her only supply was "a $15 Johnson & Johnson kit."

### Nonmedical Experience

Your experience doesn't even have to be medically related to be relevant. Many successful applicants cite nonmedical volunteer experience as evidence of their willingness to help and heal the human race. In fact, almost every one of our essayists cited having been either a volunteer or a tutor at some point in their lives.

## Developing a Strategy

Once you have decided how to incorporate the various themes into your essay, the last step is to develop a strategy—or in other words, figure out how you are going to weave your themes together into a coherent whole. Here's some advice you don't get often: don't think about this one too much. What's nice about strategy is that it tends to fall into place by itself once you develop an outline and start writing, which is what the next section is all about. So what we offer here is no more than a couple of tips for you to consider—but not to worry too much about it. In the end there really is no more we can tell you about strategy without knowing more about your personality.

### Strategy Tip 1: Keep the School in Mind

Most students write generic personal statements which are then sent to every school. That's fine, and to a degree that is expected. But it always impresses when you do your research and show in your essay why you are a good fit for that particular school (especially on supplemental applications for PA school).

"Know the schools to which you are applying and know what they look for in an applicant. Some schools are heavily research based, some only want in-state residents, some want the heaviest science preparation possible. Do your homework!"

Don't be lazy about this! You can, at the very least, find out about the school's general reputation by scanning the website (also Google, Facebook, and YouTube). Better, though, is to research the faculty and familiarize yourself with a school's specific strengths. All of this becomes fodder for the statement and will be crucial later when you are invited to interview.

### Strategy Tip 2: Keep the Rest of Your Application in Mind

Step back and take a look at your entire application package. Imagine that you are the admissions officer looking at it for the first time. What do the test scores, the science and non-science GPA, the kind of courses you took, the recommendations, the extracurriculars, and the supplemental materials say about you? Do you feel it presents a complete picture of you? If it doesn't, what can you include in your essay to round it out? Also note if there are any obvious red flags.

"If there is a hole or gap that appears in another part of the application, we will look to the statement to provide an explanation. If one is not provided, we start guessing. Anything the candidate provides is bound to be better than we hypothesize in its absence."

Also note redundancies. Don't recapitulate in your essay that which can be found elsewhere in the application. Don't repeat your GPA or your MCAT (GRE) score, no matter how impressive. And, as noted previously, don't try to cram in a prose listing of your activities and accomplishments when space is provided for you to do that elsewhere. Not only is it dull, but also shows that you don't know how to take advantage of a good opportunity to showcase your personal qualities.

### Strategy Tip 3: Avoid Discussing Medical Issues

Though known to come up during interviews, a discussion of medical issues is not often attempted in the essay and not generally advised. There are many reasons for this: (1) the essay is supposed to be about you, not about issues, (2) your audience likely knows more about the issues than you do, (3) with only two pages to do the issue justice, you will probably end up biting off more than you can chew, and (4) you risk offending someone on the committee. The natural exception to this rule is if a medical issue featured prominently in your decision to become a doctor. One essayist, for example, cites the public health care debate as one of her primary draws to the field.

Discussing your negative views of the medical field in your personal statement is an especially risky way to discuss medical issues in your essay. Like anything there are those who do it well. One of our essayists, for example, discusses what he perceives as a conflict in the medical world and demonstrates how he will contribute to the resolution of the conflict. Though he deals with what he sees as a negative conflict in the medical arena, he discusses it objectively and with tact.

Another essayist doesn't give her opinion on medical issues, but she does cite the bad experience she had with her pediatrician as a child as her chief motivation for her to do a better job as a doctor herself. Both of these examples discuss their potential roles in the resolution of the conflict. Even when you keep these tactics in mind, though, the best advice here is definitely, "when in doubt, leave it out."

### An Alternative Approach

No matter how hard and fast these rules regarding theme and strategy may seem, there will always be applicants who will decide to toss it all to the wind and take a completely different approach. The writer of one essay, for example, incorporates none of the mentioned themes into his personal statement. He doesn't talk about his motivation or qualifications for attending medical school. In fact, he only mentions medical school once, and even then it is a single reference made only as an aside. He chose, instead, to focus his entire essay on his experience as a rower at Cambridge University in England.

This is a risky approach, and one that is best taken by students with already very strong backgrounds. This applicant obviously felt confident that the rest of his application spoke well enough of his qualifications that he could focus entirely on another aspect of his life. And this approach does have the merit of painting a vivid picture of the applicant in his natural surroundings and of giving the reader a strong sense of his character and drive. Ultimately it is a personal decision. Again, the best way to gauge whether or not the risk is one worth taking is by finding a candidate capable of giving you objective and informed feedback.

# Avoiding Pitfalls

### Pitfall #1: The Hard-Luck Tale

Some truly outstanding essays are about strong emotional experiences such as a childhood struggle with disease or the death of a loved one. Some of these are done so effectively that they are held up as role models for all essays.

"I had a student who was considered a weak candidate because of poor grades and low test scores. She was African American and although she had pursued all the right avenues (classes, MCAT, volunteer experiences) to prepare herself for medical school, she remained undistinguished as a candidate—until, that is, she wrote her essay. The essay revealed her tremendous and sincere drive. She was from a crime-riddled area of NY and several of her siblings had been violently killed. She wrote about her experience and her desire to practice medicine in the city and improve the neighborhood where she was raised. It was compelling, believable, and truly inspiring."

While it's true that these poignant tales can provide very strong evidence of motivation for medical school, they are difficult to do well and need to be handled with extreme care and sensitivity. And, as we've said before, don't rely on the tale itself to carry you through—you always need to clearly show your motivation.

"This is going to sound harsh, but I don't like the tales of woe. Like the ones that begin with the mother's death from cancer. Frankly, I feel manipulated and I don't think that the personal statement is the proper mode of expression for that kind of emotion."

### Pitfall #2: Making Lists

There is a danger inherent in wanting to cram as much of your experience as possible into 500 words. The danger is ending up with what amounts to little more than a listing of your accomplishments.

"I've found that medical school applicants can have a tendency to make laundry lists…They need to take extra care to tie their interests, motivation, and preparation together and turn it into a readable and credible argument that fits them."

It is not a bad idea to include all the experience you have had somewhere in your essay. But do it in the context of a story or a personal account.

"The essay should never be merely a prose from a C.V. It's dry to read, and again, doesn't offer any additional information about the candidate."

### Pitfall #3: Excuses, Excuses

Because GPA and test scores are so important to the application process, applicants who have fallen short in either area are often tempted to use the essay to provide excuses for their poor performances. This is not always ill-advised. If there is a true anomaly in your record, the committee will look to your essay for an explanation. Applicants who do this topic well provide a brief and mature explanation of the lapse, then they spend the rest of the essay focusing on their strengths in other areas.

"Explaining a bad grade or even a bad semester can be done with finesse. I would never give staying away from that as blanket advice. But, please, just don't whine while you're doing it."

The problems come when you try to excuse a problem instead of explaining it. Some applicants, for example, try to excuse low test scores by claiming that they are not good test takers. Well, we hate to break it to them, but medical school is about taking tests. They are a large part of the curriculum and are proven predictors of academic success. So why would admitting flat-out to being a bad tester ever be a good thing? Other students try to push the blame for a bad grade onto someone else.

"Using the essay to make excuses for your overall poor record isn't a good way to get ahead. We don't need to hear about the professor who 'had a problem with you,' or how your organic chemistry professor 'wasn't from America.' These types of statements speak volumes about a person's character."

The only way to know for sure that you're not falling into this trap is to ask someone objective to proof your essay for you. Even better, find someone who doesn't even know you and ask them to describe back to you the impression they received of the writer.

## CREATING THE STRUCTURE

- Creating an Outline
- Standard Structure
- Compare and Contrast
- Chronological
- Incorporating Narrative

Now that you know what you want your personal statement to say, it is time to start writing. First, set a time limit of no more than a couple of days. The longer the time frame, the more difficult will it be to write your first draft.

The point is not to let yourself sit around waiting for inspiration to strike. As one admissions officer put it, "Some of the worst writing ever crafted has been done under the guise of inspiration."

Relieve some of the pressure of writing by reminding yourself that this is just a draft. Rid yourself of the notion that your essay can be perfect on the first try. Don't agonize over a particular word choice, or the phrasing of an idea—you will have plenty of time to perfect the essay later. For now, the most important thing is to get some words on paper.

## Creating an Outline

You are probably familiar by now with the structure of the traditional outline that you were probably taught in grade-school:

**Paragraph #1: (Introduction which contains the central idea)**
**Paragraph #2:**

- Topic sentence that ties into the central idea
- First supporting point
- Evidence for point

**Paragraph #3:**

- Topic sentence which links the above paragraph to the next
- Second supporting point
- Evidence for point

**Paragraph #4:**

- Topic sentence which links the above paragraph to the next
- Third supporting point
- Evidence for point

**Paragraph #5:**

(Conclusion which reiterates the central idea and takes it one step further)

This tried and true method is still your best bet. The problem is that it may not allow for the complexities created by the multiple themes that need to be incorporated into a personal statement. Your outline will probably end up looking more complicated than this one, but that is no excuse for not having one. In fact, the more complex the essay, the more in need of an outline it will be. Without it, your essay will lack structure. Without structure, your essay will be rambling an ineffective.

Take some time to play with the material you have, putting it into different structures, always with the goal of offering the best support for your main points. To get ideas for some different outlines that could be applied to your statement, look at some of the examples below.

## Standard Structure

The standard structure is the most common and is recommended for use in almost any circumstance. Applying it as close as you can get at this level to the simple structure outlined above. The general application of the standard structure is to introduce the themes and main points in the introduction, use the body of the text to supply one supporting point in each paragraph, and then reiterate your main points in the conclusion in light of the evidence that was presented. The following is an example of a pure standard structure used by an applicant who wanted to make the points that she was both interested in and qualified for the medical field on two levels: intellectually and from a standpoint of wanting to help people.

**Paragraph #1: (Introduction)**

**Leading sentence:** "Since my childhood, my father's inspirational recounts as a cardiologist have captured my heart and my interest."

**Summary of main points:** Introduces "two fundamental tenets" of "working to care and working to cure," noting her interest in both the academic and the caring sides of medicine.

**Paragraph #2:**

**Transition sentence:** "During my high school and college years, I have explored different areas of community service."

**First supporting point:** Interest in caring is shown through her community involvement.

**Evidence:** Tutoring geometry to high-school students and English to recent immigrants.

**Paragraph #3:**

**Transition sentence:** "I have also participated in the caring element of the medical profession, providing companionship to patients in the hospital setting."

**Second supporting point:** Interest in caring demonstrated by her hospital experience.

**Evidence:** Volunteer at several hospitals including the coronary care unit and the Cardiac Rehabilitation Center.

**Paragraph #4:**

**Transition sentence:** "It would be simplistic for me to say that I have chosen to devote my life to the medical profession only because I have a strong desire to help people."

**Second supporting point:** Also motivated by intellectual exploration.

**Evidence:** She details her passion for "[making] an intellectual leap and [managing] to land feet first upon a convincing conclusion" and describes the thrill which leaves her "thirsting for the next challenge."

**Paragraph #5:**

**Transition sentence:** "The excitement of intellectual discovery has encouraged me to explore a number of fields."

**Second supporting point:** Has a well-rounded academic background.

**Evidence:** "While my major is biochemistry, my academic interests also encompass Asian studies, languages, music, computer science, health care, and environmental policy..."

**Paragraph #6:**

**Transition sentence:** "My rewarding experiences growing intellectually have not only fueled my own passion for exploration and discovery, but have also inspired me to share my enthusiasm for learning with others, particularly in the field of science."

**Second supporting point:** Ties academic interests back to original theme of caring for people.

**Evidence:** "To help high-school students embark on their own exciting voyages to understand the world around us, I wrote a study guide describing how to approach scientific research and titled it Frontier to emphasize exploration and intellectual discovery."

**Paragraph #7:**

**Transition sentence:** "To me, there is only one profession that satisfies both my curiosity and my desire to help those in need."

**Reiteration of main points and closing sentence:** "Incorporating both the caring, personal, physician-patient relationship and the dynamism of continuous learning, the medical profession is the profession I eagerly embrace, and I believe it is also the best way I can harness my own talents and abilities for the benefit of others."

# Chronological

Another way to create an outline for your essay is by retelling the events of your life chronologically. The advantage of this approach is that it allows for a more personal approach and helps the committee to know you by turning the focus to you throughout various stages of your life. The drawback is that the points you are trying to make can get lost in the narration of your life.

The following writer uses a chronological structure beginning with the clip of an article describing him as a young boy:

**Paragraph #1: (leading Quote)**

**Leading sentence:** "One time, a family cat captured...a moth"

Provides a quote from an article describing him as a boy in 1978.

**Paragraph #2: (Introduction)**

**Transition sentence:** "This article, about me as a ten-year-old boy trying to turn a nearby drainage pond into a park, had a misprint—it was a mouse, not a moth."

Explains quote and makes main point that he was cut out to be a doctor from a young age.

**Paragraph #3:**

**Transition sentence:** "We didn't exactly live on a farm, but were in farming country."

Describes himself and his life as a boy.

**Paragraph #4:**

**Transition sentence:** "During this period, we did manage to find time for other things."

Focuses on his multiple activities throughout high-school years.

**Paragraph #5:**

**Transition sentence:** "After two semesters at Boise State, I volunteered to serve for 2 years as a missionary with the Church of Jesus Christ of Latter-Day Saints, going to the California, Ventura Mission."

Continues to college-age-years spent as a missionary.

**Paragraph #6:**

**Transition sentence:** "Returning to school, my classes included math and sciences (subjects I had shied away from before)—out of the curiosity, at first; then, to keep my options open."

Progresses his return to college and his activities and accomplishments from that period.

**Paragraph #7:**

**Transition sentence:** "In high school, I had some health problems and seen a number of doctors."

Steps back to high-school experiences to introduce theme of medicine.

**Paragraph #8:**

**Transition sentence:** "This experience soured me on the medical profession."

Interprets experiences described in last paragraph to explain late interest in medicine.

**Paragraph #9:**

**Transition sentence:** "I pursued psychology and the humanities, while growing more fascinated by health, nutrition, and what people I knew had found in 'alternative' approaches to health, including preventive and Eastern medicine."

Talks about his subsequent interest in fields peripheral to medicine.

**Paragraph #10:**

**Transition sentence:** "Upon transferring to USC, I found that my view of the medical establishment wasn't really accurate—there ARE those who care more about helping people than about the money or the intellectual pride."

Describes how his interest in medicine solidified while at USC.

**Paragraph #11:**

**Transition sentence:** "Throughout my college career, I have had to support myself financially."

Uses the transition to discuss the many jobs he has held throughout the stages in his life.

# Incorporating Narrative

Beginning your essay with a story is a common and effective method for catching and keeping the reader's interest. This is also a good way to structure your essay if you want to focus on a single event in your life. In its purest form a narrative essay does nothing but tell the story. It begins and ends with the action. This is not recommended for a personal statement, simply because at some point the connection needs to be drawn from the story to your motivation and qualifications for attending medical school.

The following are some examples of writers who have incorporated narrative into their essays. Notice how each writer provides a clear transition to the rest of their essay.

**Essay 1:** Paints a picture of herself as a child climbing into her father's dentist chair for treatment. Uses the story to transition into her desire to practice in pediatric dental care.

**Essay 2:** Begins with story of working as a deckhand for the Sea Education Association (SEA). Uses story to demonstrate teamwork skills and importance of community. Transitions from story with: "Both at sea and on land, I have found great pleasure in the rewards of upholding and enriching the worlds of which I am a part."

**Essay 3:** Tells story of her high-school teacher's battle with AIDS. Transitions with: "I entered college, believing that biology could explain to me why life's processes went awry."

**Essay 4:** Tells story of unraveling the past of a prehistoric woman by analyzing her bones. Transitions in the last paragraph with: "To a large extent, my choice to become a physician is rooted in my desire to continue to work with the human body. But I want to work with the living."

**Essay 5:** Incorporates story of his attempt to save a life aboard a train in Italy into the middle of his essay rather than at the beginning. Uses it to illustrate the lessons he learned of self-forgetful devotion and the importance of attention to detail.

Notice the variety of circumstances this type of essay can be applied to when comparing these essays. A narrative can span a lifetime or a moment. It does not have to be filled with Hollywood style action to hold interest. The briefest and simplest of events can take on meaning when told effectively. What makes all of these essays effective is their use of detail, description, and direction.

## LEADS AND ENDS

- Leading the Way
- Closing your Case

Beginnings and endings can be the most challenging part of crafting any piece of writing and, in many ways, the most important. Part of the reason that they are so difficult is that writers tend to worry about them too much. There is so much hype on the necessity of thoroughly introducing the subject and ending with sharply drawn conclusions that anxious essayists compensate by going overboard. They feel that in order to appear mature and worldly their essays must contain profound insights and sweeping observations.

Do not fall into this trap! One of the biggest complaints that our admissions officers had were essayists that tried to say and do too much in their introductions. "Just tell the story!" was repeated like a mantra in response to essayists who were trying too hard to impress. Many of these essays (not included in this chapter) would have been vastly improved had they simply removed their introductions altogether.

Do yourself a favor and forget about beginnings and endings during the first stages of writing. Just dive straight into the body of the text without bothering to introduce your themes or set the scene. The reason this technique works is that when you have finished writing the rest of your rough draft, you may discover that you don't need an introduction at all. But isn't that risky? Maybe. But believe it or not, more essays have been ruined by forced and unnecessary introductions than have been ruined by the lack of one. Largely this is because of the misconception of what an introduction is supposed to accomplish.

This is especially true if you are basing your essay around a story. It might feel risky or uncomfortable just letting the story stand on its own without being introduced first, but beginning with action is always a good idea as long as the action is tied closely into the points you are trying to make throughout the rest of the essay.

## Leading the Way

- Standard Lead
- Action Lead
- Personal or Revealing Lead
- Creative Lead
- Quotation Lead
- Dialogue Lead
- Fact Lead

The most important part of any beginning is, of course, the lead. Leads play the dual role of setting the theme of your essay and engaging the reader. The introduction should not be overly formal or stilted. You do not want an admissions officer to start reading your essay and think, "here we go again." Although admissions officers will try to give the entire essay a fair reading, they are only human—if you lose them after the first sentence the rest of your essay will not get the attention it deserves.

Just as you should not worry about your introduction until you have gotten an initial draft on paper, you should not begin writing your lead unless you are feeling inspired about a particular line. Often, you will find a good one floating around in the middle of your first draft of the essay, so don't waste time worrying about it until you have the bulk of your essay on paper.

There are many different kinds of effective leads. All of the examples below were taken from the essays in our database.

## Standard Lead

Standard leads are the most common leads used. A typical standard lead answers one or more of the six basic questions: who, what, when, where, why, and how. They give the reader an idea of what to expect. A summary lead is kind of standard lead that answers most of these questions in one sentence. The problem with this kind of lead is that, although it is a logical beginning, it can be dull. The advantage is that it sets your reader up for a focused and well-structured essay. If you live up to that expectation, the impact of your points is heightened. They are also useful for shorter essays when you need to get to your point quickly.

"Initially, my interest in medicine was due to my family."

"I am interested in participating in the Harvard M.I.T. Division of Health Sciences and Technology Program (HST) in the context of an M.D./Ph.D. to prepare for a career in medical research."

"My work experiences—ranging from public health projects in rural Latin America to work at Urban battered women's shelters to peer counseling on a college campus—reflect my concern for people's 'health' in a broad sense of the word."

## Action Lead

This lead takes the reader into the middle of a piece of action. It is perfect for short essays where space needs to be conserved or for narrative essays that begin with a story.

"The car swerved to the left."

"She dropped the box on the table and left the room because she didn't want to watch."

"It was opening night. I was about to walk on stage as Ruth in 'The Pirates of Penzance'."

"As the rusted-out Land Rover made its way cautiously through the dense thicket and cervices in the rocky dirt road, those of us sitting on top were able to peer through the trees at a sublime West African landscape."

"One day in the summer after my graduation from high school, my grandfather took me up to the attic of his house to show me something he thought would be significant for me."

## Personal or Revealing Lead

This lead reveals something about the writer. It is always in the first person and usually takes an informal, conversational tone:

"I was not in control of my life and I was miserable."

"Since my childhood, my father's inspirational recounts as a cardiologist have captured my heart and my interest."

"I decided that I wanted to be a doctor sometime after my 4-month incarceration in Columbia Presbyterian Children's Hospital in the winter of 1986-87, as I struggled with anorexia nervosa."

## Creative Lead

This lead attempts to add interest by being obtuse or funny. They can leave you wondering what the essay will be about, or make you smile.

"The melody starts slow, a quiet whirring sound of violins slowly envelopes the hall."

"The beating of an African healing drum resonates throughout all corners of the Catholic church during the weekly five o'clock student mass."

"When I consider my life experiences, I imagine them as a system of bones and joints, interconnected, cooperative, and form-giving."

## Quotation Lead

This type of lead can be a direct quotation or paraphrase. It is most effective when the quote you choose is unusual, funny, or obscure, and not too long. Choose a quote with a meaning you plan to reveal to the reader as the essay progresses. Some admissions officers caution this kind of lead because it can seem like you are trying to impress them or sound smart. Do not use a proverb or cliché, and do not interpret the quote in your essay. The admissions committee is more interested in how you respond to it and what the response says about you.

"Dr. Lewis Thomas described medicine as 'The Youngest Science' because insightful discoveries in basic research have led to the revolutionary innovations in clinical therapy that have improved the quality of life."

"One day you will read in the National Geographic of a faraway place with no smelly bad traffic. In the green pastured mountains of Fotta-fa-Zee everybody feels fine at a hundred and three 'cause the air they breathe is potassium-free and because they chew nuts from the Tutt-a-Tutt Tree. This gives strength to their teeth, it gives length to their hair, and they live without doctors, with nary a care'—Dr. Seuss, You're Only Old Once."

"I love the way he makes me laugh."

## Dialogue Lead

This lead takes the reader into a conversation. It can take the form of an actual dialogue between two people or can simply be a snippet of personal thought.

"Power ten, next stroke! shouts the coxswain over the speaker system."

"Kathy, do you believe in las brujas?"

"Peter, the woman we're about to meet will receive her first palliative treatment today."

"Why on Earth do you want to study in Africa?"

## Fact Lead

This lead gives the reader a fact or statistic that is connected to the topic of your essay or simply provides a piece of information about yourself or a situation.

"Every doctor remembers his first patient."

"In communist Hungary in 1986 ownership of property meant certain things."

"On the corner of 168th street and Broadway in New York City, there always seems to be a line of people."

# Closing Your Case

The final sentence or two of your essay is also critical. It must finish your thought or assertion, and it is an important part of creating a positive and memorable image. Endings are the last experience an admissions officer has with your essay, so you need to make those words and thoughts count. A standard close merely summarizes the main points you have made.

Some examples of standard closes include:

"But most of all, I know that for me to bring meaning to the years of instruction my professors and textbooks have given me, I must give back to the community. I have chosen to do that by becoming a doctor."

"As a lifelong commitment to society, the medical profession most completely encompasses my career goals and moral values."

"In the future, I see myself as the pedodontist whose office will be filled with excited children who climb into my chair feeling as comfortable as I always did in my father's."

"Reminiscing about how Mr. M pulled the brown marshmallow from his chopstick, I am thankful to my campers and students, their families, and my friends for helping me to affirm that this is the path I wish to follow."

If you have introduced a clever or unusual thought in the first paragraph, try referring back to it in your conclusion. The aim is for the admissions officer to leave your essay thinking, "That was a satisfying read," and "I wish there were more."

One essayist, for example, closes with:

"The once bewildered 7-year-old at the scene of an accident now has the skills and maturity to do more than change diapers; she aspires to read the film of the broken humerus or to set the cast someday soon."

The writer's reference to the bewildered 7-year-old relates back to her opening story about a car accident from her youth. This stylistic touch wraps the essay up nicely and shows that time was spent in planning and structuring.

## WRITING THE ESSAY

- Paragraphs and Transitions
- Word Choice
- The Verb Test
- Sentence Length and Structure

## Paragraphs and Transitions

Paragraphs are the pillars of the essay—they uphold and support the structure. Each one that you write should express a single thought and contain a beginning, a middle, and an end. And again, this holds true whether you are writing a traditional or a creative essay.

The first sentence of every paragraph (after the first, which is called the lead) plays the important role of transitioning. An essay without good transitions is like a series of isolated islands; the reader will struggle to get from one point to the next. Use transitions as bridges between your ideas.

As you move from one paragraph to the next, you should not have to explain your story in addition to telling it. If the transitions between paragraphs require explanation, your essay is either too large in scope or the flow is not logical. A good transition statement will straddle the line between the two paragraphs.

The transition into the final paragraph is especially critical. If it is not clear how you arrived at this final idea, you have either shoe-horned a conclusion into the outline, or your outline lacks focus. You should not have to think too much about consciously constructing transition sentences. If the concepts in your outline follow and build on one another naturally, transitions will practically write themselves. To make sure that you are not forcing your transitions, try to refrain from using words like "however," "nevertheless," and "furthermore."

If you are having trouble transitioning between paragraphs or are trying to force a transition on to a paragraph that has already been written, it may be indicative of a problem with your structure. If you suspect this to be the case, go back to your original outline and make sure that you have assigned only one point to each paragraph, and that each point naturally follows the preceding one and leads to a logical conclusion. This may result in a kind of "back to the drawing board" restructuring, but try not to get frustrated. This happens to even the most seasoned writers and is a normal part of the writing process.

## Word Choice

Well-structured outlines, paragraphs, and transitions are important parts of a solid essay. But structure isn't everything. An essay can be very well organized with balanced paragraphs and smooth transitions and still come across as dull and uninspired. The most important thing you can do to make your essay more interesting is add lots of colorful details about your life. The second most important thing you can do is pay attention to word choice.

**Rule #1:** Put your thesaurus away. Using a thesaurus won't make you look smarter, it will only make you look like you are trying to look smarter.

**Rule #2:** Focus on verbs. Keep adjectives to a minimum. Pumping your sentences full of adjectives and adverbs is not the same thing as adding detail or color. Adjectives and adverbs add description, but verbs add action—and action is always more interesting than description.

One of the admissions officers on our panel advises using the following test to gauge the strength of your word choice.

## The Verb Test

Choose a paragraph from your essay and make a list of every verb you have used. Compare your list to the one given in Table 6.2.

These are lists of the first 10 verbs found in two essays in our packages. One list was taken from our admissions team's favorite essays. The other is taken from one of their least favorite. Can you guess which is which? The essays were not being graded on verb use, obviously, and yet the correlation between strong verbs and high scores is undeniable. Think of it this way: if you had to choose an essay based solely on the verb list, which one would you rather read?

## Sentence Length and Structure

Another way to analyze the strength of your writing is to examine the pacing of your sentences. This is a good time to read your essay out loud. As you read, listen to the rhythm of the sentences. Are they all the same length? If each of your sentences twists and turns for an entire paragraph, try breaking them up for variety. Remember that short sentences have great impact.

**Table 6.2.** List of Verbs

| Column 1 | Column 2 |
| --- | --- |
| Said | Has met |
| Contorted | Can say |
| Complain | Know |
| Learned | Are usually |
| Spreading | May have heard |
| Sprang | Are |
| Strained | Is |
| Gripped | Strive |
| Had been living | May not be involved |
| Had attended | Try to perform |

One way to determine if you are using variety of different sentence lengths is to put S, M, or L (for short, medium, and long) above each sentence in a paragraph. A dull paragraph can look something like this:

M M M L M S S S M L

On the other hand, an interesting paragraph may look more like this:

S L M M L S

## FINAL TOUCHES

- Take a Break
- Revise
- The Hunt for Red Flags
- Proofread
- Read Out Loud
- Get Feedback!

Writing is not a one-time act. Writing is a process, and memorable writing comes more from rewriting than it does from the first draft. By rewriting, you will improve your essay—guaranteed. There is no perfect amount of drafts that will ensure a great essay, but you will eventually reach a point when your confidence in the strength of your writing is reinforced by the thoughts of others. If you skimp on the rewriting process, you significantly reduce the chances that your essay will be as good as it could be. Don't take that chance. The following steps show you how to take your essay from rough to remarkable.

## Take a Break!

You have made it through the first draft, and you deserve a reward for the hard work. Before you do anything else—take a break! Let it sit for a couple of days. You need to distance yourself from the piece so you can gain objectivity. Writing can be an emotional and exhausting process, particularly when you write about yourself and your experiences. After you finish your first draft, you may think a bit too highly of your efforts—or you may be too harsh. Both extremes are probably inaccurate. Once you have let your work sit for a while you will be better able to take the next (and final!) step—proofreading.

# Revise

- Substance
- Structure
- Interest

Once you have taken a break away from your essay, come back and read it through once with a fresh perspective. Analyze it as objectively as possible based on the following three components: substance, structure, and interest. Do not worry yet about surface errors and spelling mistakes, focus instead on the larger issues. Be prepared to find some significant problems with your essays and be willing to address them even though it might mean significantly more work. Also, if you find yourself unable to iron out the bugs that turn up, you should be willing to consider starting one or two of your essays from scratch, potentially with a new topic.

Use the following checklist to critique the various parts of your essays.

## Substance

Substance refers to the content of your essay and the message you are sending out. It can be very hard to gauge in your own writing. One good way to make sure that you are saying what you think you are saying is to write down, briefly and in your own words, the general idea of your message. Then remove the introduction and the conclusion from your essay and have an objective reader review what is left and do the same. Compare the two statements to see how similar they are. This can be especially helpful if you write a narrative, to make sure that your points are being communicated in the story.

Here are some questions to ask regarding content:

- Have you answered the question that was asked?
- Is each point that you make backed up by an example?
- Are you examples concrete and personal?
- Have you been specific? Go on a generalities hunt. Turn the generalities into specifics.
- Is the essay about you? (The answers should be "Yes!")
- What does it say about you? Try making a list of all the words you have used to describe yourself (directly or indirectly). Does the list accurately represent you?

- Does the writing sound like you? Is it personal and informal rather than uptight or stiff?
- Read your introduction. Is it personal and written in your own voice? If it is general or makes any broad claims, then have someone proofread your essay once without it. Did they notice that it was missing? If the essay can stand on its own without it, then consider removing it permanently.

## Structure

To check the overall structure of your essay, do a first-sentence check. Write down the first sentence in every paragraph in order: Read through them one after another and ask yourself the following:

- Would someone who was only reading these sentences still understand exactly what you are trying to say?
- Are all your main points addressed in the first sentences?
- Do the thoughts flow naturally, or do they seem to skip around or come out of left field?

Now go back to your essay as a whole and ask yourself these questions:

- Does each paragraph stick to the thought that was introduced in the first sentence?
- Is each point supported by a piece of evidence?
- Are all of the paragraphs of roughly the same length? When you step back and squint at your essay do they look balanced on the page? If one is significantly longer than the rest, you are probably trying to squeeze more than one thought into it.
- Does your conclusion draw naturally from the previous paragraphs?
- Have you varied the length and structure of your sentences?

## Interest

Many people think only of mechanics when they revise and rewrite their compositions. But as we know, the interest factor is crucial in keeping the admissions officers reading and in making your essay memorable.

Look at your essay with the interest equation in mind: personal + specific = interesting. Answer the following:

- Is the opening paragraph personal? Do you start with action or an image?
- At what point does your essay *really* begin? Try to delete all the sentences before that point.
- Does the essay "show" rather than "tell?" Use details whenever possible to create images.
- Did you use any words that you wouldn't use in a conversation? Did you take any words from a thesaurus? (If either answer is yes, get rid of them.)
- Have you used an active voice?
- Did you do the <u>verb check?</u> Are your verbs active and interesting?
- Have you overused adjectives and adverbs?
- Have you eliminated trite expressions and clichés?
- Does it sound interesting to you? If it bores you, it will bore others.
- Will the ending give the reader a sense of completeness? Does the last sentence sound like the last sentence?

## The Hunt for Red Flags

How can you know if you are writing in a passive or active voice? Certain words and phrases are red flags for passive voice, and relying on them too heavily will considerably weaken an otherwise good essay. To find out if your essay suffers from passivity, go on a hunt for all of the following, highlighting each one as you find it (Table 6.3).

When you are done, how much of your essay is highlighted? You do not need to eliminate these phrases completely, but ask yourself if each one is necessary. Try replacing the weak phrases with stronger ones.

## Proofread

When you are satisfied with the structure and content of your essay, it's time to check for grammar, spelling, typos, and the like. There will be obvious things you can fix right away: a misspelled or misused word, a seemingly endless sentence, or improper punctuation. Keep rewriting

**Table 6.3.** Passive Voice

| | | |
|---|---|---|
| Really | I hope | For instance, |
| There is | Maybe | Very |
| It is essential that | Usually | In fact |
| Nonetheless/ nevertheless | Have had | I believe |
| In conclusion | Rather | Can be |
| Yet | It is important to note that | Perhaps |
| Although | However | May/may not |
| I feel | In addition | Somewhat |

until your words say what you want them to say. Ask yourselves these questions:

- Did I punctuate correctly?
- Did I eliminate exclamation points (except in dialogue)?
- Did I use capitalization clearly and consistently?
- Do the subjects agree in number with the verbs?
- Did I place the periods and commas inside the quotation marks?
- Do I keep contractions to a minimum? Are apostrophes in the right places?
- Did I insert the name of the proper school for each new application?

## Read Out Loud

To help you polish the essay even further, read it out loud. You will be amazed at the faulty grammar and awkward language that your ears can detect. It will also give you a good sense of the flow of the piece and will alert you to anything that sounds too abrupt or out of place. Good writing, like much music, has a certain rhythm. How does your essay sound? Interesting and varied, or drawn out and monotonous. Reading your essay out loud is also a good way to catch errors that your eyes might otherwise skim over while reading silently.

## ALWAYS Get Feedback!

We've mentioned this point many times throughout this chapter, but it can never be emphasized enough: get feedback! Not only will it help you see your essay objectively, as others will see it, but it is also a good way to get reinspired when you feel yourself burning out.

You should have already found someone to proof for general style, structure, and content. If you have to write multiple essays for one school, you should also have had them evaluate the set as a whole. Now, as the final step before submitting your application, find someone new to proof for the surface errors that will only be seen with fresh eyes. Copy this page and have them check off the questions as they proof.

And, as we said earlier, if you are having trouble finding someone willing (and able) to dedicate the time and thought that needs to be put in to make this step effective, you may want to consider getting a professional evaluation. IvyEssays offers a number of different <u>editing services</u>. Whether you are looking for <u>quick feedback or a full edit</u> we have an option for you.

## FUNNY MISTAKES

**(AKA See what happens when you don't proofread)**
You would be amazed at the things that get written into admissions essays—even at the top schools. The following is a list of some of the funniest mistakes found by the admissions officers on our team. Remember that behind the hilarity of these errors lurks a serious message: always proofread your essays! Otherwise you will get the same reaction that these other applicants did: "It makes you wonder if these kids care about their essays at all," said one of our staff. "I never know whether to call it apathy or ignorance," said another "but either way the impression is not good." But then again, at least they laugh!

- Mt. Elgon National Park is well known for rich deposits of herds of elephants.
- I enjoyed my bondage with the family and especially their mule, Jake.

- The book was very entertaining, even though it was about a dull subject, world war II.
- I would love to attend a college where the foundation was built upon women.
- The worst experience that I have probably ever had to go through emotionally was when other members of PETA (People for the Ethical Treatment of Animals) and I went to Pennsylvania for their annual pigeon shoot.
- He was a modest man with an unbelievable ego.
- Scuba One members are volunteers, but that never stops them from trying to save someone's life.
- Hemmingway includes no modern terminology in a *Farewell to Arms*. This, of course, is due to the fact that it was not written recently.
- I am proud to be able to say I have sustained from the use of drugs, alcohol and tobacco products.
- I've been a strong advocate of the abomination of drunk driving.
- If Homer's primary view of mortal life could be expressed in a word it would be this: life is fleeting.
- Such things as divorces, separations and annulments greatly reduce the need for adultery to be committed.
- It is rewarding to hear when some of these prisoners I have fought for are released, yet triumphant when others are executed.
- Playing the saxophone lets me develop technique and skill which will help me in the future, since I would like to become a doctor.
- However, many students would not be able to emerge from the same situation unscrewed.
- I look at each stage as a challenge, and an adventure, and as another experience on my step ladder of life.
- "Bare your cross," something I have heard all my life.
- There was one man in particular who caught my attention. He was a tiny man with ridiculously features all of which, with the exception of his nose, seemed to drown in the mass of the delicate transparent pinkish flesh that cascaded from his forehead and flowed over the collar of his tuxedo and the edge of his bow tie.
- Take Wordsworth, for example; every one of his words is worth a hundred words.

- For almost all involved in these stories, premature burial has a negative effect on their lives.
- I know that as we age, we tend to forget the bricklayers of our lives.
- I would like to see my own ignorance wither into enlightenment.
- Another activity I take personally is my church Youth Group.
- The outdoors is two dimensional, challenging my physical and mental capabilities.
- Going to school in your wonderfully gothic setting would be an exciting challenge.
- My mother worked hard to provide me with whatever I needed in my life, a good home, a fairly stale family and wonderful education.
- I hope to provide in turn, a self-motivated, confident, and capable individual to add to the reputation of Vasser University whose name stands up for itself. [Note: the correct spelling is Vassar.]
- Filled with Victorian furniture and beautiful antique fixtures, even at that age I was amazed.
- They eagerly and happily took our bags, welcomed us in English, and quickly drove us out of the airport.
- Do I shake the hand that has always bitten me?
- In the spring, people were literally exploding outside.
- Freedom of speech is the ointment which sets us free.
- I first was exposed through a friend who attends [school].
- As an extra, we even saw Elizabeth Taylor's home, which had a bridge attaching it to the hoe across the street.
- *Name of Activity:* Cook and serve homeless
- *On a transcript:* AP English
- *Misspelled abbreviation on another transcript:* COMP CRAP (computer graphics)
- *Handwritten on an interview form under Academic Interests:* Writing.

# [CHAPTER 7]

# The Interview (Part One): It's not about you, it's about them

$C$ongratulations! You've made it to the interview phase of the PA school application process and your chances for getting accepted have increased dramatically. A typical PA program receives a thousand or more applications for a precious 25 to 50 slots each cycle. Your chance of acceptance at this point is roughly 2½% to 5% for any given program. Many programs invite approximately 200 applicants to interview, and if you're invited to interview, your chances have now increased to 12½% to 25%; much better odds. Your job now is to claim your seat in the upcoming class by being the most prepared applicant in the room that day. You've taken control of your situation and rather than be one of the thousand faceless drones trying to break into the PA profession, you've decided to do more...be more! At last, you're not just making positive steps in the way you interview, you're making positive steps toward getting accepted!

So go ahead and pat yourself on the back, you've worked hard to get here and you deserve to be very proud of yourself. This is just the beginning; however, not the end. You now have to take all of the knowledge and expertise I provide you and reduce it into a condensed, manageable format within the framework of the questions and answers that you will be asked. You may feel a bit anxious and overwhelmed at this point, but trust me, I'm going to break all of the knowledge I present in this chapter into easy to digest, bite-sized nuggets of valuable information that will make you the perfect PA school applicant.

Coming into the home stretch, I'll show you how to really supercharge your entire interview using targeted answers to questions you will encounter during a PA school interview. You will discover how using the PA program's various web properties (program website, Facebook, YouTube, Blogs, etc.) to uncover the qualities and multipliers (more on this later) that will set you apart from everyone else. This is the most important part of my tailoring method, and ultimately the technique that has helped me become the pioneer in coaching thousands of PA school applicants to success.

I'm going to teach you how to infuse these qualities into your answers in order to tailor your responses to the program you are interviewing with. In this chapter, I'm going to take you to another level. A level that only the *perfect applicants* can reach. I will be referring to the perfect applicant a lot in this chapter.

I want you to think of the PA school interview process similar to studying for a test in school. In order to pass the test, you need to study the material to be most prepared. Imagine knowing the answers to the questions on that test before taking it? Well, I'm going to provide you with the questions and answers. And not just carbon-copy answers. I'm going to show you how to tailor your answers relative to the specific PA program that you are interviewing with. This book is the secret weapon you need to blow away the competition and get accepted into the PA school of your choice.

In this chapter I've compiled the most commonly asked questions that you may be asked, along with examples of qualities and multipliers that you can use to supercharge your responses. *The answers to the questions I provide are only examples, not to be memorized verbatim.* You will need to do the work and dig deep to find the qualities and multipliers for each program you interview with, in order to find out what they value most. Additionally, the answers I supply are just suggestions. The answers I provide are amazing answers with my proven methodology behind them, helping to guide them to be solid answers that the admissions committee will want to hear...but they're not necessarily 100% the right answers for you. This is a guide, use it to mold your own answers based on your personal experiences, qualities, and values. Don't memorize the answers in this chapter, you will come off as fake and unnatural at your interview. Use this chapter as a springboard to help you rise above the competition and make a favorable impression on the admissions committee.

In addition to samples of the most common questions and answers, I'm also providing you with the most common DOS and DON'TS for each question, which will provide you with some additional insight and make answering the question much easier.

Remember it's tailoring the interview to the program you are interviewing with that is the most important thing.

## BEFORE THE INTERVIEW

Okay, now that you are pumped up thinking about how much you're going to learn in this chapter, it's now time to go to work! I'm going to break this section down into five easy-to-manage segments:

- General Preparation
- Types of Interviews
- Dos and Don'ts for the PA School Interview
- Dealing with Anxiety
- Final Preparation

Okay, let's get started!

## GENERAL PREPARATION

You've done all of the work necessary to get your CASPA application completed, and submitted. You wait in anticipation to hear back from the PA programs you applied to, and then one day you open your email and see that your top choice PA program has sent you a response. You hold your breath, your heart starts pounding, and you quickly click to open it up. You read, "Congratulations, we would like to extend you an offer to come interview at our PA program." After you jump up and down, call your friends, and soak up the moment, it's now time to prepare for the final, and most difficult, piece of the PA school application process. Your job has just begun.

You should be very proud of yourself for a job well done. Go out and celebrate, then be ready to come back and do the work of preparing for your PA school interview.

You look great on paper, but now it's time to prepare to show the admissions committee that you look the part in person too. That means you must begin preparing for your interview long before you stand tall before the admissions committee.

The sooner you complete the work, the sooner you can start reviewing these example questions and answers and preparing your own responses. Don't procrastinate, get it done ASAP!

## Sleep Hygiene

If you are used to keeping erratic hours, going out with your friends to late in the morning, or just not getting the recommended 8 hours of sleep per night, now is the time to get on a regular sleep schedule. This will enable you to be fresh every day, and have the energy to do the upcoming work necessary to give the performance of your life-time on the day of your interview.

## Take Care of Yourself

If you don't already exercise, start slowly with an exercise routine that will energize you on a daily basis. What is the best exercise? The one you'll do! Cut back on your caffeine use. At this point, you should be on a natural "high" anyway. Start eating a healthy diet, low in sugar and high in protein. Get your body running like a well-oiled machine and by the time your interview comes, you'll be happy, healthy, and confident.

The night before the interview, be sure to arrive to your hotel early (if you're traveling). I strongly recommend that you do a "dry run" and either walk, or drive, to the exact location of the building, and room, where you will be interviewing the next day. Check out the traffic conditions and the length of time it will take you to get there. Anticipate the worst-case scenario, and leave early in the morning. You can always go to a restaurant for a small breakfast if you have a lot of spare time. Don't forget to carry the phone number of the program, just in case you hit a traffic jam, or for some unforeseen reason, you are going to be late.

Be sure to eat well the night before your interview. Have a light dinner, and don't eat anything that may linger on your breath. Absolutely no alcohol that night. You certainly don't want to smell like you just came from the bar before your interview.

Take out your suit (yes, wear a suit!), shirt/blouse, belt, socks, and shoes. Try everything on BEFORE the interview. Make sure everything looks impeccable; shoes shined, no stains on your clothes, and place everything in a space where you don't have to go searching for any items in the morning. You will be nervous enough and you don't need to be frantically searching for your belt for 15 minutes on the morning of your interview.

Next, take 15 to 20 minutes sitting quietly in your room. Close your eyes, and visualize your entire interview. See yourself impeccably dressed, confident, answering all of the interview questions with ease. This technique is powerful, and it's used by many professional athletes before a big game. A basketball player may visualize herself making every shot she takes, stealing the ball on defense, and grabbing rebound after rebound. This is the equivalent of doing a dry run in your mind.

I always advise bringing a small mirror with you to the interview. You may want to take a close look at your face, teeth, hair, etc. immediately before entering the interview room. Sometimes PA programs offer food and drinks during the course of the day. Having mustard on your face, or a piece of broccoli caught between your teeth will certainly not score you any points. And believe me, I've seen it all.

## The Day of the Interview

Set your alarm clock to go off early, and ask the hotel front desk to provide you with a wake-up call as a backup. Have a small breakfast before getting dressed. Take a good look in the mirror, and keep your jacket on a hanger while traveling to the interview. Be sure to check yourself again in the bathroom mirror once you're ready to go. Do not overdo the perfume or cologne, and please, no nose rings, tongue rings, or bright pink hair. Now is not the time to "express yourself."

I recommend that you arrive at least 15 minutes early; no sooner, no later. If you are very early, sit in the car or a restaurant, and practice your answers to the questions I will prepare you for. Some applicants like to meditate to calm the nerves. Others like to make phone calls to some of their friends, or a significant other in order to get some moral support.

DO NOT bring a cell phone into your interview. You will be too tempted to check text messages, or perhaps sneak in a phone call. Even worse, you don't want your cell phone to ring (or vibrate) in the middle of your interview.

Be sure to greet everyone at the program as if they are evaluating you, and have a decision on your outcome. If you say the wrong thing to the receptionist, she is likely to pass on this negative experience to one of the committee members that she works with every day, and that will not help your chances. Be friendly, and smile at everyone.

## Silence your Inner Critic

When you walk into your interview and meet the other applicants (the "competition"), your inner critic inside of your brain may start telling you, "You're not good enough," "These other applicants seem more qualified than I am," "I don't belong here." The inner critic can be your worst enemy in this situation and you need to know how to silence it. A very simple technique is to say "Stop" in your mind each time a negative thought enters it. Do this 20 times if you have to. Eventually, the negative thoughts will quiet down and you'll be able to focus on the task at hand. I will teach you a technique to help you with anxiety later in the chapter.

Think about the fact that you would not be here if you didn't have what it takes. Your application was screened by the admissions committee, and they selected you for an interview. You have what it takes, so focus on that. Everybody in that room has an equal chance. However, if you use the quality and multiplier techniques, you will be much more prepared than anyone else.

Additionally, when you walk in and meet the other applicants, be the first one to extend a handshake and introduce yourself. If an applicant walks in after you arrive, do the same. Do not allow yourself to be intimidated by the applicant who is going to boast about his medical experience, GPA, or the fact that he's already been accepted to another program. Keep the conversations light, and cursory. If necessary, walk into a quiet corner and focus on the task at hand.

## TYPES OF INTERVIEWS

Many of you will have no idea what to expect when showing up for your PA school interview. I'm not just talking about the questions and answers; I'm talking about the various types of interview formats that you may encounter during this critical phase of the application process. Each program utilizes a format to assess you as an applicant, depending on what values and qualities they look for in the applicant. You must prepare for each of these formats in order to give a peak performance. Let's take a look at the most common formats that you may encounter.

## The Solo Interview

The one-on-one interview is the traditional interview format. Your solo interview is typically conducted by a high-level program faculty member.

This member is going to have a critical role in the decision-making process, so it goes without saying that you must be at the top of your game. **The solo interviewer will have a key set of qualities and traits that she is looking for, and this is your chance to show her how perfectly you match what she is looking for.** Once you finish reading this chapter, you will feel very comfortable in this traditional interview format. Before you know it, you'll be trying to see where your seat is located in the classroom. The best way to do this is to follow the steps I've laid out for you in this chapter with perfectly tailored answers (more on this later).

## The Panel Interview

Imagine walking through the door and there are three smiling faces staring back at you (or maybe not smiling?). This interview format is certainly a bit more anxiety provoking, but not to worry. There are several reasons why a program uses the panel interview format, but the main reason is to eliminate any bias that one interviewer may have toward an applicant. It also ramps up the pressure a little bit on the applicant, allowing the interviewers to see how well you handle pressure and deal with authority.

To relieve some of the pressure and be prepared for this interview format, try to find out beforehand if a panel interview is on the agenda, how many people will be on the panel, and get their names if possible. If the program provides the names of the interviewers, be sure to do some research and find out as much information about each member. Perhaps one of them won a specific award, or was past president of the American Academy of Physician Assistants (AAPA). Maybe you went to the same college as one of the members, or you both played the same sport. Also, be prepared for the panel to change members on you. Perhaps the three people you've researched conducted an interview with the first applicant of the day, but the panel switches out with three other members for *your* panel interview. Don't panic! As long as you've read this book and prepared your own answers to the most common questions, you'll be fine.

One suggestion I have—no, one **strong recommendation**—is to make **eye contact with each member on the panel.** For instance, if the interviewer on the left asks you a question, begin answering the question by making eye contact with her for 5 seconds, then adjusting your gaze to the middle interviewer for 5 seconds, and next to the interviewer on the right for 5 seconds. Repeat this process until you've fully answered the question. It is very important to engage everyone at the table, or you risk alienating one of the committee members who may develop a subconscious resentment toward you. (More on this in the next chapter.)

One applicant told me that she was in a panel interview, and one of the interviewers got up in the middle of the session, took a seat behind her, and started asking her questions from a position behind her back. Perhaps this is a technique to see how you handle stress. If this happens to you, remember that eye contact is the key to gaining credibility and trust. So turn your chair *sideways,* and look to your left or to your right so you can establish eye contact with everyone.

## The Multiple Applicant Interview

In my opinion, this is one of the most stressful interviews you will face. You're sitting in a room with other applicants who want *your* seat in the program. Don't worry, I'm going to give you some sure-fire techniques to help ensure your voice is heard and you stand out from the crowd in a favorable way. The multiple applicant interview is a great opportunity to showcase your ability to interact well with others, and also allows the committee to see if you'd be a good "fit" for their program. This is a great thing for you if you are well prepared utilizing the techniques I've shown you in this chapter. Think about it, you'll be in a room full of applicants that aren't using qualities and multipliers as part of their responses, and you will certainly stand from the rest of the applicants.

PA programs love teamwork; it's a trait that is absolutely necessary if a class is going to gel and help each other through an intense program. This type of interview is a great way for the members to see if you *play well with others.* Are you going to be a team player willing to help others, or a loner who can't be bothered by students who may be having difficulties? This group interview is not a time to be passive or shy. You want to be assertive, but not aggressive. The interview should create a win-win situation. This is a time to be balanced in your approach. You don't want to be the person who says nothing, and appears to be intimated by the other applicants. On the other hand, you don't want to be the aggressive, chatty, know-it-all who thinks he will score high by dominating the competition and not allowing them the time to speak. If you want to ace the multiple applicant interview, show your leadership skills by knowing when to speak and when to listen. If someone gives an answer to a question, perhaps you can interject by saying, "I think Sally makes a good point, and I might add..." Do not use the word, "but," because it really means you don't agree with Sally.

# The Multiple Mini Interview (MMI)

A multiple mini interview consists of a series of short, structured interview stations used to assess noncognitive qualities, including cultural sensitivity, maturity, teamwork, empathy, reliability, and communication skills.

Prior to the start of each mini-interview rotation, candidates receive a question/scenario and have a designated period of time to prepare an answer. For instance, there may be a card on the wall or door for you to read a scenario. You may have 3 minutes to read the scenario, then enter the room and have 7 minutes to give your answer.

Upon entering the interview room, the candidate has a short exchange with an interviewer/assessor. In some situations, the interviewer observes while the action takes place between the applicant and an actor.

At the end of each mini-interview, the interviewer evaluates the candidate's performance while the applicant moves to the next station. This pattern is repeated through a number of rotations. The questions asked are usually situational questions that touch on the following:

- Ethical decision making
- Critical thinking
- Communication skills
- Current health care and societal issues

Although participants must relate to the scenario posed at each station, it is important to note that the MMI is not intended to test specific knowledge in the field. Instead the interviewers evaluate each candidate's thought process and ability to think on her feet. As such, there are no right or wrong answers to the question posed in an MMI, but each applicant should look at the question from a variety of perspectives.

# The Student Interview

The student interview usually consists of two or three first- or second-year students, asking you questions in a more relaxed format. But don't be fooled by the conversational nature of this interview. The students will have a say on whether they like you or not, particularly evaluating you as someone they would like to have as a classmate. **Treat the students with the utmost respect. Look at this interview as a great opportunity to let them sell you on why you should attend their program.**

You are not likely to be asked traditional interview questions in the student interview, but if you've followed the guidance in this book, you'll be prepared to discuss qualities and multipliers that you've researched before the interview. Be sure to visit the student society website, or blog, to find out what special events or projects that the students are involved with. Students are very proud of their program and the events they participate in. Perhaps a group of students went on a mission trip to South America to provide vaccinations to children in isolated regions of a country. It would be really nice to know this information ahead of time. Take the time to do your homework and let the students know that you have the same values and qualities as they have.

## DOS AND DON'TS FOR THE PA SCHOOL INTERVIEW

Now that you know how to prepare for the various PA school interviews you may encounter, let's take a list of DOS and DON'TS.

**DO:** Your homework (research). Learn everything you can about the program(s) where you will be interviewing. Start early. The program's website is the first place to start. Leave no stone unturned. View every page and link on the site. Don't forget about social media, either. Check out the program on Facebook, Google, Blogs, Student sites, and YouTube. For example, I found the following about the Barry University PA Program using Google:

> No More Tears Charity Golf Tournament (1)
> by Barry University PA Program
>
> EVENT DETAILS
>
> A group of motivated, <u>civic-minded</u> Barry University Physician Assistant Students have committed to raising money and awareness for the No More Tears Project. No More Tears' is a 100% not-for-profit organization that is operated entirely through the <u>selfless</u> efforts of volunteers and donors whose <u>mission is to rescue the victims of domestic violence and human trafficking</u>.

**How many applicants do you think will know about this effort come interview day? Can you infuse these qualities into some of your answers**

to interview questions at Barry? The qualities are underlined, and the multiplier is the Event (No More Tears Charity Golf Tournament).

DON'T: Continuously call the program and become a nuisance. Don't ask questions that you should know from searching the program's website.

DO: Invest in a new suit if you don't have one. You may be able to rent a suit also. The point is, always lean toward overdressing rather than underdressing.

DON'T: Come to the interview with nose rings, tongue rings, flashy jewelry, low-cut blouses, unkempt hair, or a wrinkled outfit. Dress for success. You want the focus to be on you, and not your attire.

DO: Eat a simple, well-balanced meal the night before your interview—and a good breakfast the morning of.

DON'T: Eat a bunch of spicy food, or junk food, the night before your interview. You don't want to have acid reflux first thing in the morning which will make you feel miserable. Do not drink alcohol before your interview to calm your nerves. I will teach you a much better way to deal with anxiety later in the chapter.

DO: Get a good night's sleep the night before.

DON'T: Stay up all night stressing over the interview, or cramming information into your brain. Reassure yourself that you are prepared, watch a movie, and relax as best you can.

DO: Take a shower, brush your teeth, and spend the time to look your best. As you'll see in the next chapter, the visual component of an interview will weigh significantly on your score.

DON'T: Smoke before your interview; your clothes will smell of tobacco and being a smoker is not the best way to show that you are an advocate for health.

DO: Arrive early to your interview, review your notes, and practice the anxiety-relieving technique that I will teach you in the next section.

DON'T: Be rude to *anyone* you meet at the program, including the other applicants. For example, if the receptionist asks you, "Did you have any trouble finding us?", your response should be: "Absolutely not, you gave excellent directions, thank you." You want to start things off on a positive note.

DO: Be a real person. In other words, do your best to be likeable, trust-worthy, and credible.

DON'T: Panic. Remember, it's not about *you*, it's about them. Get out of your own head and shut off that inner critic. You are prepared for this interview. Remember that the committee wants you to solve their problem—finding the perfect applicant who has all of the qualities *they* are looking for.

Here is a technique to quiet your mind and relieve the anxiety that you are likely to feel on the day of your interview.

# DEALING WITH ANXIETY

As soon as you open your eyes on the morning of your interview, I can assure you that your heart will start racing, your breath will be shallow and rapid, and you will probably have a knot in the pit of your stom-ach. Don't panic! What you're experiencing is healthy anxiety. Your body's physiology is acting appropriately. The challenge is to avoid panicking.

As an example, think about the following situation: You come out of your friend's house and begin walking to your car. You suddenly hear loud barking and a huge dog, foaming at the mouth, is making a B-line right toward you. Your physiology begins to go into fight-or-flight mode; your pupils immediately dilate, your breathing becomes rapid and shallow, and your heart rate goes through the roof. I think it's safe to say that at a time like this, it's not exactly the best moment to figure out your taxes. So if you want to be able to think clearly, particularly on the day of your inter-view, you need to control your physiology, because you're likely to be in fight-or-flight mode when you enter the building.

If you are not prepared for this on the day of your interview, your plan is to "wing it." This plan is going to cause a lot more anxiety, and you will be in the fight-or-flight mode throughout the entire interview process. You will have a very difficult time answering interview questions if you can't change this physiological response quickly.

## The SHIELD Technique

Dr. Eva Selhub, a mind/body expert, resiliency coach, motivational speaker, and an executive coach, teaches a powerful technique used to instantly reduce a person's stress and anxiety level. Her technique is to put up your SHIELD.

You can use this technique while waiting to be called into the room, and nobody will have to know that you're using it.

The acronym stands for:

Stop

Honor the feeling

Inhale

Exhale

Listen

Decide

Author of *The Love Response* (2), Dr. Selhub promotes a simple philosophy: At its best, stress motivates. At its worst, stress annihilates. Good leaders motivate. Bad leaders annihilate.

The choice is yours to decide how stress will influence your leadership.

If you find yourself in an anxiety-provoking or stressful situation (like the PA school interview), you can use the SHIELD™ technique to instantly change your physiology.

As a result, if you utilize this technique, your breathing will slow down, your heart rate will decrease, your pupils will return to normal size, and you will be able to think much more clearly.

Here is how the technique works:

> Once you feel your anxiety level becoming too high, *stop* what you are doing. Then, ***honor the feeling***. Ask yourself: are you anxious, afraid, frustrated, angry, lonely, or tired? Next, ***inhale*** and ***exhale***, 10 times in a row. (When you breathe in, imagine filling an empty balloon in your belly with your breath. When you breathe out, imagine deflating the balloon). Repeat the breaths 10 times, and you will notice a soothing, calming effect. By this time, your adrenaline is dropping, and you will be able to think clearly and focus on the task at hand. So, ***listen*** to your mind and become aware of your thoughts and feelings now. Finally, ***decide*** to do something different than ruminating, which is counterproductive. Now, your body is out of fight-or-flight mode.

You can repeat the above technique as many times as necessary to help you relax and focus.

## Silencing the "Inner Critic"

In a variety of stressful situations, we become our own worst enemy. I can remember arriving for my interview at Yale and meeting all of my "competition." Everyone in the room had a master's degree, except for me. My inner critic came alive. "I'm never going to get in!" I was being very hard on myself and extremely judgmental. Negative self-talk only serves to perpetuate the anxiety and make things worse.

Here are some things *your* inner critic may shout at you on the day of your interview:

- "I should have prepared more."
- "Everyone here is more qualified than I am."
- "I'll never get accepted."
- "I'm a loser; I don't belong here."
- "I'm going to blow this interview."

Don't wait until your interview to address your inner critic. Here are some steps that you can take to deal with your inner critic weeks or months before your interview:

1. *Monitor your thoughts.*

   Becoming aware of your inner critic's voice—if you will—is the first step. You can achieve this by simply being mindful of those thoughts. Just notice when and where the thoughts occur, and then write them down on a piece of paper or in a journal.

   You may become acutely aware of certain patterns in your thinking. Once you master being mindful and get the negative thoughts on paper, you can begin to silence the inner critic.

2. *Notice your judgments.*

   Instead of making judgments, try describing your thoughts or feelings. For example, you may be having a conversation with a fellow student about a class you are both taking. You may really like the professor, and in the course of the conversation, you might say, "Professor Jones is a great teacher." Your classmate might not agree with you and say, "I think he's a terrible teacher." Both of you are making judgments and probably putting the other person on guard to defend his or her decision.

   If you said instead, "I appreciate that Professor Jones always comes prepared to class. It makes it easier for me to stay focused."

You are not being judgmental; you are simply describing the way you *feel* about him. Nobody can dispute that, not even your friend.

The point is that when we are being judgmental, especially of ourselves, we promote more intense feelings of negativity. And at the interview, we want to stay positive.

3. *Challenge your automatic negative thoughts.*

   Feelings aren't facts! Once you practice mindfulness and become good at documenting your thoughts (judgments), it is time to challenge those negative thoughts with the facts. You may feel like you don't have what it takes to be accepted, but if you look at the facts, you may change your mind.

   For example, if you were to review your CASPA application, you would see that you've worked hard to complete the requirements for PA school. The fact that you received an offer to interview means that you've already beat out several hundred applicants to get the interview. So although you may certainly feel like you don't have what it takes to get accepted, the facts prove otherwise.

   Try to challenge all of your negative thoughts with the facts. Chances are you will find that you are beating yourself up for no reason.

4. *Practice, not perfection.*

   The goal of practicing mindfulness and keeping your judgments in check is to achieve awareness and make gradual changes. Becoming aware of the problem is the first step. However, if you are in denial about how your judgments and negative thoughts affect your mindset, you will not be able to make any progress at all. It takes constant vigilance to achieve improvement with being mindful.

5. *Reevaluate your values.*

   Make sure that whatever you are beating yourself up over is worth striving for. Some goals, like kindness, integrity, and being self-disciplined, enhance the meaning and quality of life, whereas others only feed into your sense of defectiveness. Some people think, *If I only went to a better school, I'd have more self-esteem.* By the way, the best way to increase self-esteem is to do estimable things!

## FINAL PREPARATION

Remember, your goal at the interview is to help the interviewers' job become a little easier by showing them that you have the qualities and values they're looking for in a perfect applicant. It's not about you, it's about them. Your interviewer is not out to trip you up. She's a regular person, with a family, worries, and insecurities just like you. In fact, she may be just as nervous as you are.

Be prepared for multiple interviews. I recommend that you call the program beforehand to see if they will tell you how many interviews you will have, and perhaps even who will be your interviewers. Find out if they use traditional questions, behavioral questions, or a multiple mini interview (MMI) format.

From the time you enter the building, until the time you exit the building, you are being evaluated. Maintain a professional appearance and persona throughout the entire process. Greet everyone with a smile and a handshake, from the Dean of the program, to the janitor vacuuming the floors. Remember that although you may only be there for one day, these people spend 40 hours a week together, just like in any other job. They're like a small family, and they've seen a lot of candidates come and go. If you say something negative or controversial in front of the receptionist, don't be surprised if she passes that information on to the committee members. You've done too much work to be here, it would be a tragedy to be rejected because you insulted one of the staff.

Finally, be sure to treat the student interviewers with the utmost respect. Don't let your guard down because you think they don't have much of a say with respect to scoring your interview. Take advantage of the opportunity to let them tell you what they like most about the program. As I'll mention in another section of this chapter, above all else you want to be likeable.

## THE TAILORING METHOD

In this next section, I'll introduce you to a powerful tool that will help you leave the competition in the dust: the tailoring method. I will also explain the idea of the perfect applicant. More importantly, I'll finally introduce the most important pieces to the "interview question puzzle," the qualities and multipliers.

If you've read any of my books, you've probably noticed that I do things a little differently than anyone else. As the pioneer in PA school applicant coaching, and author of four books dedicated to helping PA school applicants, you know that I use specialized techniques and training to help applicants get accepted! There are many more PA school coaches available to PA school applicants now than when I started in 1996; however, none have the longevity, experience, and knowledge that I've gained over the past 20 years working with applicants from all over the country. Yes, I help applicants get accepted!

Okay, so what is my secret? How have I been able to help so many applicants succeed, where others have failed on their own in the past? Because there is one key to success that I teach those I coach:

"It's not about you, it's about them!"

You may *think* it's about you. After all, you really have a strong passion to become a physician assistant; you've completed all of the prerequisites for PA school, you have a 3.7 science GPA, 3,000 hours of hands-on medical experience, phenomenal GRE scores, and excellent references. You're now ready to "strut your stuff" at the interview.

But it's really not about you. It's about meeting the needs of the program and demonstrating that you have exactly what they are looking for in a perfect applicant. The interviewer(s) look to see if you have the qualities to become a great student and a great PA. More importantly, do you have what it takes to be a good classmate, complete the rigorous program, pass your boards, and be a respectable representative of their program out in the community.

Many other PAs, friends, coworkers, and PA school coaches will tell you that the best thing you can do at your interview is summarize your past experiences and highlight your personal strengths and accomplishments. And to be honest, when those strengths and experiences are better than the other applicants, it's often enough to get accepted.

This is not my philosophy. This is the "old school" way of interviewing. What if you don't have a clear-cut advantage over the other applicants? In the huge applicant pool, there will be the best of the best at the interview, and *everyone* will have a strong resume.

What if you sit across from the interviewer(s) and go on and on about your accomplishments, thinking you are the perfect applicant, not knowing that what you're saying is irrelevant to what the interviewer(s) and the program are looking for in a strong applicant. It's not about you, it's about them.

The program knows exactly the type of applicant they're going to accept long before you enter the interview room. Many of the interviewers have been doing this for a long time. They instinctively know the qualities and traits the program desires. They obviously don't know the specific name of the applicants they are going to accept, but take my word for it, they know the type of person they want and more importantly, they know the strengths (or qualities) that this person MUST possess.

The question now becomes, how do you become that person the program wants to accept? How do you demonstrate the qualities that the program values most?

You must point out ways you can be of value to the program: how you can help them achieve *their* goals, based upon your past training and experience. You'll get your reward if they invite you to join the upcoming class. But be more interested in them than you are in yourself. Be there for them. Take it from my own experience being on an admissions committee; it's a tough job, so help them make the right decision.

For starters, point out ways you can be of value to the program: how can you help them achieve their goals based upon your past training and experience?

But how does one do this?

By using the tailoring method of course!

So, by now it should be clear that the program you are about to interview with already knows the type of applicant they want to accept. I refer to this person as the perfect applicant.

## The Perfect Applicant

You are going to see this term a lot in this chapter, because it is my goal to turn you into this person before you step into the interview room.

What is a perfect applicant? As mentioned above, every program already has the kind of person in mind they want to accept into their program. The person will need to *demonstrate* at least two or three of the qualities the program values or emphasizes based on your research. When the program is conducting interviews, the person who best reflects these qualities is the one who is going to score the highest at the interview. This person is the perfect applicant.

Here is a simple formula to remember if you want to be the perfect applicant:

$$PA = (A + Q)^m$$

To better understand this formula, I'm going to break down the components for you.

A = Answer

Simply stated, the A in the equation is the answer you provide to the question the interviewer asks you. **Ideally, this will be a success story from your past, one that clearly demonstrates an example of you succeeding in your past jobs, or any other relevant scenarios.**

It's always a good idea to go into every interview prepared with a few of these success stories at your disposal. Everyone can draw a blank when asked a question at an interview. If you have a few of these success stories to fall back on, you can avoid that awkward silence that occurs when you draw that blank.

Q = Qualities

**Qualities are what make up the perfect applicant.** These are generally different types of knowledge, skills, or abilities that the program considers to be of paramount importance. If you want to set yourself apart in the interview, these are the things you need to reference or exemplify in your interview.

As mentioned above, the interviewer(s) will have a set of qualities in mind that the perfect applicant must have. It is your job to find out what these qualities are and demonstrate to the interviewer that you possess them. I'll show you how to find those qualities in the next section. I'll also show you how to infuse these qualities into your answer.

## Example Qualities

| | | |
|---|---|---|
| Accountability | Adaptability | Ability to handle stress |
| Assertive | Academic ability | Analytical thinking |
| Attention to detail | Balanced | Collaboration |
| Cooperation | Confidence | Compassion |
| Caring | Discipline | Diversity |
| Empathetic | Energy | Ethical |
| Friendly | Humility | Hard working |
| Knows when to ask for help | Leadership | Life-long learner |
| Listener | Maturity | Proactive |
| Problem solver | Service oriented | Strong interpersonal skills |

<u>m = multipliers</u>

Multipliers are the "icing on the cake" in your interview, or a supercharger or booster for each of your answers. Multipliers are nuggets of information that you can bring up in your interview that the interviewer is not expecting you to know. Generally speaking, this would include things like special programs, initiatives or events, volunteer programs, to name a few. The *m* acts as an exponent because it really increases your chance of being the perfect applicant exponentially!

The reason multipliers are so effective is that they help you demonstrate your level of knowledge of the program and their culture, and really makes a statement about the amount of preparation you've done.

**Using multipliers has the ability to make you look like you're already a student in the eyes of the interviewer.**

I'm going to show you how to find multipliers in the next section.

I hope that makes sense to you as a PA school applicant. Let's again review the idea of the equation:

$$\text{Perfect Applicant} = (\text{Answer} + \text{Question})^{\text{multiplier}}$$

When the interviewer asks you a question at your PA school interview, they will be expecting you to respond. You have a choice. You can give them a straight, literal, carbon-copy answer that is your best attempt at giving them the information they need, or you can utilize the tailoring method by using the perfect applicant principle above. Answer your question by infusing your response with a quality (A + Q) that the program is looking for in a qualified applicant, and then put the icing on the cake by including a multiplier (m).

The truth is your competition won't stand a chance if they are simply using the "old school" interview techniques.

So obviously, the next question is:

How do I find the specific qualities that the program is looking for?

This is the key, because you can't simply guess which qualities you *think* the program values. You have to know exactly. If you try to be clever and emphasize a quality that the program doesn't value you're just going to sound like every other, vanilla, applicant who interviews that day.

Our goal is to have you rise to the top of the applicant pool, so let me show you how to identify which qualities your program values, and at the same time, it will reveal how to find some of the multipliers that are like an added bonus!

# Finding Qualities and Multipliers

It is absolutely essential to respond to interview questions by infusing the program's desired perfect applicant qualities into your answers. The next step is to figure out what these qualities and multipliers are AND where they can be found.

Preparing for the PA school interview process has changed dramatically over the years with the proliferation of technology, namely the internet. In the old days, we had to request program brochures, attend the open house, and call the program and ask questions. Research was limited to speaking with graduates of the program, purchasing a hard copy of the old PA Programs Directory, printed information from the AAPA, or from your state (constituent) chapter of the AAPA. This was all cursory information that was available to everyone else; no "top secret" stuff. Everyone walked into the interview on an even playing field.

Times have changed, however. Information on PA programs can be found everywhere on the internet. With the explosion of the internet comes an explosion of information available to PA school applicants at your fingertips, and all you have to do is complete your homework and take advantage of this information.

Brochures have been replaced with websites for every program. Using photos, videos, and other multimedia, programs are now able to give prospective applicants a glimpse into their culture, mission, and values. Even before you walk into the interview room, you will have a good idea of what it will be like to attend their program.

But that's not all.

They also leave clues. What kind of clues? The kind of clues that are very interesting to me, and from now on, will be very interesting to you. Beginning with the program's website, this is where we begin to dig around for potential qualities and multipliers, the life-blood of the tailoring method and perhaps the most influential part of a successful PA school interview.

You may be thinking, "Looking on the program's website is not exactly a revolutionary idea..." You know what? You'd be surprised how many of the applicants I coach thought the same thing at the beginning.

But it's not just about gathering some background information on the program or simply studying their mission and values before heading into your interview. When I tell you that PA programs are leaving clues on their website, I mean it. One of the absolute best places to discover the types of qualities that their perfect applicant must possess is their website, and this is how you do it.

## 1. General Information

Begin by going to the program's website and **get a good feel for all of the general information that is available,** including:

- History of the program
- Longevity of the program
- First-time pass/fail rates on the PANCE
- Location
- Any recent news items
- Cadaver lab
- International clinical rotations
- Class size
- Learning style of the program; problem-based learning?

These are just the basics! None of this information is going to set you apart from your competitors, but you will sure set yourself apart (the wrong way) if you don't know this stuff inside and out. The point is you need to **get a feel for the culture of the program, what they value most, any current events or volunteer work the students participate in, or any news stories relevant to the program.**

Notice any themes that may jump out at you. I have found that occasionally, qualities and multipliers can be found among the general information, depending on how much information the program chooses to present on their website. For example, you may get a sense that the program values "diversity," and "working with underserved populations." Take note of anything the program is going out of its way to share.

## 2. Finding Qualities

**Once you have a solid understanding of the general information, the next thing you need to do is "drill down" to get some more interview-focused information.** This is where the social media pages, student blogs, Google, and student society pages usually come into play.

Be sure to read the "About Us" link, then check the other internet resources mentioned above. You'd be surprised to see what pops up from doing a simple Google search of the program.

Make sure to read the mission statement thoroughly. The program will usually tell you specifically what types of applicants they prefer. Sometimes they look for students who come from diverse backgrounds, sometimes they look for in-state applicants who want to stay and work in the state after graduation, and sometimes they generally publish that they are looking for applicants to work in underserved areas after graduating.

What does this mean for you, the interviewee? This is a *crucial* step. As I mentioned earlier in the chapter, you absolutely need to tailor your answers to the program you are interviewing with, and you do this by infusing your answers to their questions with qualities and multipliers.

I pulled these qualities from the Duke University PA Program Home Page:

We value:

- Diversity and inclusion
- Integrity
- Excellence
- Professionalism
- Team work and respect
- Kindness and compassion
- Scholarship

You will notice that Duke has hinted how important it is to find applicants with diversity as their top listed value. Therefore, it is important that you are able to demonstrate that you possess this quality. If you cannot demonstrate this quality, pick one of the others where you can provide an example of how you've demonstrated that quality.

How do you do this?

By carefully choosing to infuse your answers with this quality identified above. The quality is underlined in the following answer.

### "Why are you interested in attending Duke's PA Program?"

"There are some obvious reasons why I want to attend Duke. Duke is the birthplace of the physician assistant profession. Duke has a ninety-nine percent first-time pass-fail rate on the PANCE over the past five years. I know if I attend this program I will be well prepared to pass my boards and become a certified PA. This program is consistently ranked as one of the top-ten PA programs in the country by U.S. News & World Report. The program has been accredited

> since 1972, and I know that if I attend this program I will benefit from a strong curriculum and from well-established clinical rotation sites."
>
> "I've been very selective in the programs that I've decided to apply to because I want to attend a program like Duke where I can add value. I'm focused on a program that truly values diversity; something I'm extremely passionate about. I know that there is a rich migrant community established in the area and I will have the ability to help patients from diverse backgrounds." (Second-year student blog: Katherine Caro, January 29, 2016)

Now keep this in mind. A program can reveal their desired perfect applicant qualities in many different ways. You can find qualities in videos. You can find them on blog posts. You can find them on Facebook. The point is you really have to dig around to see what you can turn up. Trust me, it's in your best interest!

In the Question and Answer portion of this chapter, I'll show you examples of how to tailor your responses to the program(s) you are interviewing with using qualities.

## 3. Finding Multipliers

The way to find multipliers on the program's website is not unlike searching for qualities. The home page is certainly the place to get started.

> The PA Program is committed to recruiting and matriculating a wide range of students including but not limited to those who are underrepresented in the PA profession because PAs interact with patients, families, and communities from diverse backgrounds.

The multipliers are not something that will necessarily be as obvious. Why? Well, mainly because many of the interviewers don't even know that multipliers exist. Rather, they don't expect you, the interviewee, to zone in on them and like a ninja, and use them as a secret weapon in your interview.

As I mention before, **multipliers are like the "cherry on the top" of your interview answer. This is really where you get to separate yourself from everybody else at the interview.** So focus on the programs upcoming (or past) events, special programs that they offer or any outreach programs or initiatives they support.

Here is a sample multiplier from a second-year PA student's blog entry at Duke.

### Second-Year Student Blog: Katherine Caro

"One of the aspects that attracted me to the Duke Physician Assistant Program was the program's commitment to fostering an environment that encourages students to serve their community. This commitment was something I noticed immediately on my interview day while learning about various opportunities afforded by the program including the <u>Underserved Community Scholar Program."</u>

"I was able to help many Latino families because of the rich migrant community established in the community."

Bringing up this multiplier (*Underserved Community Scholar Program*) in your response really shows that you have done your research, but in reality, gives the interviewer the feeling that you are "already one of them." You bridge the gap between being an applicant and a student by showing your level of comfort and understanding with the way the program does things. Using the same question as above, see the new answer with the quality underlined and the multiplier highlighted in bold.

### "Why are you interested in attending Duke's PA Program?"

"There are some obvious reasons why I want to attend Duke. Duke is the birthplace of the PA profession. Duke has a ninety-nine percent first-time pass-fail rate on the PANCE over the past five years. I know if I attend this program I will be well prepared to pass my boards and become a certified PA. This program is consistently ranked as one of the top-ten PA programs in the country by U.S. News & World Report. The program has been accredited since 1972, and I know that if I attend this program I will benefit from a strong and reputable didactic program, and from well-established clinical rotation sites.

I've been very selective in the programs that I've decided to apply to because I want to attend a program like Duke where I can add value. <u>I'm focused on a program that truly values diversity; something I'm extremely passionate about.</u> **I also have a great deal of experience working with underserved communities and Duke's Underserved Community Scholar Program will allow me to continue to do so while still in school.**"

## Final Thought on Qualities and Multipliers

Everything said and done, finding qualities and multipliers on a program's website is not especially difficult. As long as you take the time to really explore the website, making sure to "leave no stone unturned," you will be sure to find the qualities and multipliers you need to position yourself as the perfect applicant.

However, the program's website is not the only place that a program will reveal its qualities and multipliers. For example, Google, "Emory PA Program Special Events," and see what you find. You will find that the class of 2015 PA students are rehabilitating a home for Habitat for Humanity during orientation week, August 2013. You replace "Emory PA Program" with any program you choose in your Google search.

# QUESTIONS AND ANSWERS

Okay, here's the section you've been waiting for: the questions you're going to be asked at your interview. I am going to present a few samples from each interview format so you can get an idea of how to answer questions using qualities and multipliers. I will provide a list of many other questions that you will likely be asked at your interview, and I will provide you with a blueprint to help you find and document your own qualities and multipliers for each program.

## Traditional vs. Behavioral Questions

Most interview questions fall into two broad categories, with some slight overlap. The two categories are traditional interview questions and "behavioral" or "competency"-type questions.

Traditional questions are the most commonly asked questions at a PA-school interview. They are also the easiest to prepare for since almost every PA program asks similar questions in this format.

Traditional interview questions allow the interviewer to get a feel for:

- your knowledge of the PA profession
- your reasons for choosing the PA profession
- your personality
- your seriousness as an applicant (are you just testing the water, or are you a serious candidate?)
- your communication skills
- your interpersonal skills
- your fitness for the program

There is an art and a science to conducting a great interview. A great interview goes beyond the traditional questions that one would expect and uses various techniques and styles to extract information from the candidate. As a PA you will have to think on your feet and work under stressful conditions. The admissions committee wants to know if you have what it takes to make it through school and be a good ambassador for their program once you graduate.

More and more PA programs are utilizing a technique called *behavioral interviewing*. Interviewers can interpret what you say about yourself and your past behavior as an indicator of how you will behave in the future.

As you probably know from watching the multitude of crime dramas on television, someone with a history of criminal activity becomes a prime suspect. Once someone is shown to have broken the law, it is statistically likely that he or she will do it again at some point.

You are a "prime suspect" for acceptance into the PA program's upcoming class. The committee is looking to see how you've responded to situations in the past, which can help them predict how successfully you will respond to similar situations that may occur when you're a practicing PA.

It's in your best interest to be able to demonstrate through the use of recent, relevant examples that you have done similar jobs with proven success. When the interviewer begins to see patterns and hear about successes in your past experiences, you will be considered a serious candidate for admission.

Behavioral questions can really catch you off guard if you are not used to them and have not prepared for them. They require a lot more thinking than traditional questions. "How do you handle stress?" (a traditional-type question) is a lot easier to answer than "Tell me about a time when you had to handle a stressful situation."

Because behavioral questions are a bit more touchy-feely than traditional questions, they seem to be inviting you to open up and be more of a human personality to the interviewer. This is not a time, however, to bare your soul.

Behavioral questions may even seem like trick questions, because they definitely require you to do some thinking and might even require some soul-searching. You need to prepare ahead of time for these questions, otherwise you're going to start rambling and the committee is not going to understand what you are talking about. Don't try to "wing it" with these type of questions.

As mentioned above, behavioral questions can be a set up for you to give too much information. Don't become flattered by the interviewer's interest, or you're going to give way too much information and stray away from the actual question. "It's interesting that you asked how I handle stress. I am thinking about learning a meditation technique, Transcendental Meditation (TM), to help me learn to relax on a daily basis and get more in touch with my feelings."

Uh-oh!

That's why I'm here to help you not look like a phony. I want to give you a heads up on the kinds of questions you may encounter during your interviews, both behavioral and traditional, and to help you craft some model answers and get you thinking about how you can tailor your response using your own experiences and frameworks.

When I help applicants prepare for an upcoming interview via my mock interview coaching service, I've come to realize how many applicants are actually "winging it" out there. Studies show that those who do mock interviews before the actual interview, outperform applicants who don't do a trial run, hands down.

I'm also going to present you with some absolute "no-no's" to look out for. I'll give you some outlines and structure in which you can fit *your* specific information and come off like a professional interviewee, no matter what kind of question is thrown at you. I'll provide you with clues as to what the interviewer is really getting at with her question and how to successfully navigate the dark waters. I'll also provide you with guidance on what *not* to do.

Keep in mind this mantra; "it's not about you, it's about them," when preparing your answers to interview questions. If you don't learn anything else from this chapter, this mantra will help you quite a bit. As I mentioned, I'm going to give you special training in being prepared for interview questions, but I'll also provide you with everything else you need to succeed at your PA school interview. Your competition won't stand a chance!

As you'll see in the answers I provide for you, I have underlined the qualities that the answer requires. You should now be familiar with what the qualities are and their importance in the tailoring process. The qualities are underlined.

Also, don't forget about the multipliers: the extra bits of information that will supercharge your answers. They will be highlighted in bold.

I will also provide a list of "DOS" and DON'TS" at the end of each answer.

Before we start this section, I want to make it very clear to you that **these answers are a guide and not meant to be memorized. Use the sample answers as a tool, but you still have to do the work!**

## THE TRADITIONAL QUESTIONS

### "Tell me about yourself"

Chances are very likely that you will be asked this traditional question at your interview, and trust me, the committee doesn't want to know that you love to meditate on the beach at sunrise, or that you're an avid runner. What they're really asking is, why are you a good fit for our program?

Your answer to this question can greatly influence the outcome of your interview. The interviewer(s) wants to know that you have the necessary qualities to fulfill exactly what they're looking for: the "perfect applicant." If you've done your homework as mentioned above, you will know exactly the core must-haves to be accepted to this program.

When answering this question, you'll want to weave a story that explains how your experiences and skill sets have led you to the PA profession, and this program in particular. Show them that you have the qualities they're looking for.

Here is a good answer that will help guide you and help you build your own responses.

#### Example Answer

I think the best way to do that would be to tell you about a time when I was faced with a pretty serious situation while working as an EMT. In order to keep current on procedures and protocols, our squad held 4-hour training sessions on Saturdays. Because our supervisor was trying to squeeze too many topics into one session, we all felt overwhelmed and anxious because we weren't able to absorb all of the information in that short period of time. Everyone expressed concerns, but nobody came up with a solution. Because training is so important to EMTs, I came up with a solution. I suggested we use our Saturday training sessions to cover one topic at a time. I suggested that we break down the individual topics into one every Saturday, for 3-month blocks of time. Everyone was thrilled with this idea, and we were able to provide an enhanced learning capacity and reduce the stress and anxiety in the squad. I bring this story up because I think it highlights two things I pride myself on: solving problems and thinking outside of the box.

Qualities: problem solver and thinking outside the box

DOS:
- ✓ Focus on the strengths that the program is looking for.
- ✓ Keep the story succinct and to the point.
- ✓ Keep the story focused on work accomplishments.

DON'TS:
- ✗ Don't talk about your love for hiking or your passion for playing tennis.
- ✗ Don't stray.
- ✗ Don't focus on personal situations, keep it focused on work accomplishments.
- ✗ Don't recount any situation that occurred over 10 years ago.
- ✗ Don't talk about educational or work experiences that are not relevant to being a strong PA school applicant.
- ✗ Don't open your answer by giving your name and where you are from.

Another way to answer this question would be to incorporate the following dialogue in your answer:

*I have been in the _____industry/field for the past___ years. My most recent experience has been_____ _____ in the _____industry/career field. One reason I particularly enjoy this job, and the challenges that go with it, is the opportunity to connect with people/patients. In my last/current job I formed some significant patient relationships resulting in a deeper understanding of what it takes to be a competent medical provider.*

*My real strength is my ability to _____.*
*I pride myself on my reputation for _____.*
*When I commit to_____, I make sure_____ _____.*

*What I am looking for now is a profession that values diversity, _____, and_____, where I can use my qualities and strengths to become a competent physician assistant.*

### "Why should we select you?"

This is a very common PA school interview question; "Why should we select you over the other applicants interviewing today?" What makes you unique? The interviewer(s) will usually tell you how competitive the applicant pool is this year and that they have a lot of qualified applicants to choose from. You might feel a little disheartened at this point, but don't let it get to you. If you weren't one of those highly qualified applicants, you wouldn't be there. The committee simply wants you to convince them that you have what it takes to be a god fit for their program.

Your goal at the interview is to claim your seat and to show the committee that you are the solution to their problem: finding the best applicants.

### Example Answer

> I believe that I am uniquely qualified to attend Stanford's PA program because of your program's mission to have its graduates focus on primary care in California, and to work in underserved communities. I also know that it is important at Stanford to increase the enrollment and deployment of under-represented minorities. As you can see from my CASPA application, I have several years of hands-on medical experience working in underserved communities, and it seems to me that the **Stanford Medical School's Free-Clinics** that offer quality health care to underserved populations is incredible. There are so many PA programs that desire applicants to work in underserved areas, but few of them provide the opportunity to do this on campus. My experience working with underserved populations prepares me to hit the ground running in this program.

Quality: desire to work in underserved areas
Multiplier: Stanford Medical School's Free Clinics

DOS:
   ✓ Show you understand the mission of the program because you have researched their website.
   ✓ Your research on the program before going to the interview may show you how you can best "fit in" with the culture.
   ✓ Show that you have experience working in underserved areas, that you don't just talk-the-talk, you walk-the-walk.

DON'TS:
   ✗ Don't mention that you have spoken with the other interviewees that morning you feel that you are the most qualified.
   ✗ Don't brag.
   ✗ Don't be afraid to reiterate portions of your CASPA application that show you fit their needs.
   ✗ Don't bring up working in underserved areas if you have no experience doing so. Choose a different quality to focus on.

## "What is your greatest weakness?"

Please do not say that you are a perfectionist or any other of those faux weaknesses that can be turned into strengths. And certainly don't tell them that you're an alcoholic, but you are now in recovery. (If they hand you a rope, don't hang yourself with it.) This is a serious question that requires a serious answer. The committee actually wants to know what areas you've struggled with and what you've done to overcome these shortcomings. To answer this question appropriately, you will have to do a great deal of self-reflection. We all have weaknesses and turn them into positives that work for us, it shows adaptability as well as insights into our character—two desirable traits to have as a PA student.

Beware, they also may be looking for flaws that fit a pattern of those applicants who may have dropped out of the program in the past.

### Example Answer

I have a tendency to be a great starter and a poor finisher when it comes to writing papers. I've learned a different approach to dealing with this issue. For example, when writing papers in college, I would always leave the most difficult, time consuming research for last, which led to procrastination and anxiety. Now, I've learned that I do much better when I tackle the difficult research first, while I have the most energy, and leave the less time-consuming research until the end, so I won't feel so burdened to complete the paper. I break the project into smaller goals, and set a deadline for achieving each one. I know as a student in this program, there is no time for procrastinating. Students cannot afford to fall behind in classwork. I pride myself on being able to examine problems and come up with strategic solutions.

Qualities: self-aware, problem solver

DOS:
- ✓ Turn a weakness into a strength.
- ✓ Spend some time reflecting on a legitimate weakness you've identified and how you overcame it.
- ✓ Make sure you let them know that your weakness never gets in the way of your performance, and that you know how to strategically correct problems when they do arise.

DON'TS:
- ✗ Don't tell the committee that you walk on water and have no weaknesses.

✗ Don't use a cliché, faux weakness that can be turned into a strength.

✗ Don't hang yourself; now is not the time to talk about your alcoholism, arrest record, or the fact that you are a loner.

### "What are your goals as a PA?"

This question can be a trap to see if you plan to actually work in a primary care setting, working with underserved populations, or if your goals are inconsistent with the program's mission. To make this question easy to answer, I advise that you break the goals down into short-term, medium-term, and long-term goals.

### Example Answer

I have short-, medium-, and long-range goals once I become a PA. My short-term goal is to work, clinically, in the primary care setting with underserved populations. I wish to build on what I've learned in PA school and solidify a strong foundation in medicine that will help me throughout my entire career. My medium-range goal, say 5 years from now, is to work in research. I worked on a lot of research projects in college and I have a strong desire to continue doing so as a physician assistant. I notice that City College has done some groundbreaking research in areas like PTSD, Alzheimer's, and developing a new aspirin to fight cancer. I have a particular interest in finding a cure for Alzheimer's disease. My long-term goal is to tie in my clinical background, along with my research experiences, and one day teach at a PA program. I would like to give back to the profession by helping to educate and motivate students.

Quality: has specific goals
Multiplier: the groundbreaking research conducted at City College

DOS:

✓ Break your goals into short-, medium-, and long-range goals.

✓ The applicant has done his homework in researching the program. He has also tied his answer into the fact that he has a history of doing research in the past.

✓ Support your answer with a specific example found in your research that the admissions committee will not expect you to know about: their "groundbreaking research."

✓ Three acceptable scenarios to provide (for goals as a PA) in your answer include: practicing clinical medicine (working directly with patients), doing research, and teaching at a PA program.

DON'TS:

x Don't tell the admissions committee that you want to start your career in a specialty, like cardiology. This goal is inconsistent with the mission of the program and it shows that you are close-minded with respect to discovering opportunities in the other disciplines you will discover on clinical rotations.

x Don't forget to research the program before your interview.

x Don't discuss anything specific that you cannot support on your CASPA application. If you have never done research, don't tell the committee that doing research is one of your goals, unless you can provide strong justification for this decision.

## Thirty-Five Traditional Questions

1. Why do you want to become a PA?
2. Why do you want to attend our program?
3. What are your goals as a PA?
4. What do you consider your strengths?
5. How would you describe your personality?
6. What experience do you have that qualifies you to join our program?
7. What do you know about our program?
8. What do you value most in a classmate or coworker?
9. How have you stayed current or informed about the PA profession?
10. If I asked your coworkers or fellow students to say three positive things about you, what would they say?
11. If it comes down to you and one other applicant, why should we select you?
12. If we remember one thing about you, what should that be?
13. Have you applied to other programs? Which ones, and why did you choose them?
14. What is a "dependent" practitioner?
15. Why do you want to change careers (if applicable)?
16. Explain your undergraduate grades.
17. If you had a patient with a language barrier, how would you assist the patient?
18. What makes you mad?
19. Tell us something unique about yourself that's not already included in your application.

20. If you could change one thing about the PA profession as you understand it today, what would you change?
21. What do you like to do outside of school?
22. What area of medicine do you see yourself practicing after graduation?
23. Tell us your thoughts on health care reform.
24. Do you think health care reform will be a positive or a negative for PAs? Why or why not?
25. Should all PA programs be master's-level programs?
26. What is the difference between a PA and a nurse practitioner?
27. Where do PAs fit on the hierarchy ladder with nurses, nurse practitioners, physicians, and technicians?
28. Is it important for PAs to join local, regional, and national associations?
29. What do you think the most challenging part of being a PA is going to be?
30. What does integrity mean to you?
31. What is going to keep you from succeeding in this program?
32. If you could go back or forward in time and do anything either in real life, or fiction, what would you change?
33. Who inspired you the most in life and why?
34. What was the last book you read? What was the plot? Was there a hidden message?
35. Name a time when you were dependent on others.

## THE BEHAVIORAL QUESTIONS

Most PA programs now utilize behavioral questions as their preferred way to choose top candidates because they allow the interviewers to find out what specific skills, knowledge, and experience the PA school applicant possesses. What this means is that the interviewers interpret what you say about yourself and your past behavior as an indicator of how you will behave in the future.

It is in your best interest to be able to demonstrate through the use of recent, relevant examples that you have done similar jobs with proven success.

While a traditional interview includes straightforward questions like, "How do you handle stress?", the same behavioral question would be,

"Tell us about a time when you had to handle a stressful situation, and how you dealt with it." The traditional form of this question is very simple to answer: I exercise/meditate/practice yoga. The behavioral question is much more difficult and requires an example of a situation or task.

Behavioral interview questions can be immediately recognized by the wording used. Here are some examples of how a typical behavioral question may start:

- "Tell me about a time…"
- "Can you give me an example of…"
- "What was the biggest/most important/most difficult…"
- "Describe a time when…"

As soon as the interviewer begins a question in this fashion, you should immediately think, behavioral question. You will need to provide "an interview story" that highlights the different competencies and skill sets the program is looking for. The problem is that although many applicants might have a general idea of how to answer these questions, their answers usually come out way too long and unfocused, and don't put the applicant in the best light.

That's why you need to be aware of the behavioral questions you are likely to be asked, and to create stories and adapt them to relevant competencies to the attributes of a PA.

Here is a list of common behavioral-based interview question topics:

1. Teamwork Interview Questions

   If the role calls for being a team player, you will be expected to give specific examples that demonstrate you work well with others.

2. Leadership Interview Questions

   If people may be reporting to you, or if you've had to take charge of a difficult situation at a job, you will be expected to answer questions about your ability to lead and motivate others.

3. Handling Conflict Interview Questions

   The PA profession requires a lot of interaction with patients and multiple health care providers (or challenging situations with other colleagues). The interviewer may ask you for examples of how you handled or defused tricky situations.

4. Problem Solving

Being a PA requires critical thinking skills and the admissions committee may want to know about challenging issues/situations that required some innovation or outside-the-box thinking.

5. Biggest Failure Interview Questions

More and more PA school interviewers are asking failure questions. Whether you like it or not, you need to be prepared to have a good answer.

For many of you who are recent college graduates, and really have not hit the workforce yet, you may have a little more difficulty answering behavioral questions. Keep in mind that behavioral questions don't have to be related to health care or a past job. You may need to relate stories from your education, team sports, or volunteer positions. The key is to relate your answer to the qualities being sought in the question.

Here are six rules for answering behavioral questions:

1. Your answer/example must be specific.
2. Your examples should be concise; don't ramble.
3. Your examples should include the action you took.
4. Your examples must demonstrate your role.
5. Your examples should be relevant to the question asked.
6. Your stories must have results.

## Preparing for Behavioral Interviews

PA programs have a defined set of skills and "key competencies" they desire in a strong PA school applicant. These skill sets and competencies could include: decision making and problem solving, leadership, motivation, communication, interpersonal skills, critical thinking skills, the ability to work within a team, compassion, the ability to work autonomously, and the ability to influence others. In preparation for your PA school interview, research your answers to the following questions:

1. What are the necessary skills and "key competencies" programs desire in PA students?
2. What skills are necessary to be a physician assistant, or a physician assistant student?

3. What makes a successful PA school applicant?

4. What would make an unsuccessful PA school applicant?

5. What is the most challenging part of being a PA?

# The STAR Technique

A great way to answer behavioral questions is to use the STAR technique. STAR is an acronym for: The Situation/Task, the Action you took, and the Result (or outcome).

For example, you may need to recall a time when you had to work under stressful conditions (situation or task). To handle the situation, you had to organize your employees/classmates/coworkers and discuss options to achieve a goal (action). Following the plan you developed, you were able to accomplish the goal on time (result). Using the STAR technique process is a powerful way for you to frame your experiences.

Here are few tips for answering behavioral questions:

✓ Don't ramble and go off on tangents.

✓ Listen, listen, and listen! Remember, we have two ears and one mouth for a reason. If you are unsure about what the question is specifically asking for, ask for clarification. When you respond, be sure to recall your past accomplishments in detail.

✓ Practice your behavioral strategies using real-life examples. The last thing you want to do is attempt to "wing it." By practicing with real-life examples, you will be able to recall your past experiences and accomplishments with confidence at your interview.

The following information explains the STAR technique in detail:

### Situation or Task

Describe the situation you were in, or the task you were assigned to accomplish a goal. You must describe a specific event or situation, not a generalized description of what you have done in the past. Be sure to give enough detail for the interviewer to understand the scenario. The situation can be an event from a previous job or from a volunteer experience that is relevant to the question.

## Action

Describe the action you took, and be sure to keep the focus on yourself. Even if you are discussing a group project or effort, describe what *you* did—not the efforts of the team. Don't tell what you might have done, tell what you did.

## Result

What happened as a result of your action? How did the situation/task end? What did you accomplish? What did you learn?

Use examples from internships, classes, school projects, activities, team participation, community service, hobbies, and work experience as examples of your past behavior. In addition, feel free to use examples of special accomplishments, whether professional or personal, such as scoring a winning touchdown in the championship game, being elected to office in an organization, winning a prize for your artwork, surfing a big wave, or raising money for charity. Wherever possible, quantify your results. Numbers always impress committee members.

Remember that many behavioral questions try to uncover how you responded to negative situations. You'll need to have examples of negative experiences ready, but try to choose negative experiences that you made the best of—better yet, those that had positive outcomes.

Here's a good way to prepare for behavioral-based interview questions:

- Identify six to eight examples from your past experiences where you demonstrated behaviors and skills that PA school admissions committees seek.

- Half of your examples should be totally positive, like accomplishments or meeting goals.

- The other half should be situations that may have started out negatively, but either ended positively or you made the best of this outcome.

- Vary your examples. If you are a college student, examples from high school may be irrelevant. Try to use examples from the past year.

- Use the STAR technique to answer these questions.

The night before your interview is not the time to prepare for behavioral questions. You should start preparing for them long before your interview.

In the interview, listen carefully to each question, identify the question as a behavioral question ("Tell us about a time when...?"), recall a situation that you reviewed before your interview that pertains to the question being asked, and immediately think "STAR" technique.

**"Tell me/us about a time when you had to overcome obstacles to get a job done?"**

The interview committee wants to know if you can think for yourself and that you are a problem solver. "Tell me about a time..." should clue you in, immediately, that this is a behavioral question.

### Example Answer

While in college, I was involved in a group assignment where four of us had to do research on the hepatitis C virus, and prepare a presentation of our findings to faculty members and students in the science department. I was assigned to this group late in the process. During my first meeting with the group, I quickly realized that although a large chunk of the research they gathered was very thorough, it was not very useful for a presentation. The information was way too technical, and not very conducive to a PowerPoint presentation for those with no prior knowledge about hepatitis C. Rather than telling the group to start from scratch, I restructured the complex information into a simpler format. Everyone agreed with the changes and we incorporated the data into an effective PowerPoint presentation. We all received an award for our presentation. I take great pride in being able to come up with simple, effective solutions to seemingly impossible problems.

Quality: problem solver

DOS:
- ✓ Take a moment to brag a bit. This is a time to show off your problem-solving skills, but don't go overboard.
- ✓ The applicant took what could have been a disastrous research project and turned it into an award-winning presentation. Rather than starting over from scratch, she looked at the data already collected and revised it into a much simpler format that the audience would be able to digest and understand.
- ✓ This answer lets the interviewer know that she can think outside of the box and is a creative problem solver.

DON'TS:

    ✗ Don't tell a story where you solved all of the world's problems.

    ✗ Don't over exaggerate your accomplishment.

    ✗ Don't take credit for something you didn't actually do.

**"Tell me about a time when you had to handle a stressful situation?"**

This is a very common question that you must be prepared to answer. The interviewer is looking for a specific example of a stressful situation you've had to face and how you resolved it. He may also want to see what you consider stressful.

### Example Answer

I started a new job as a medical assistant in a family practice. After working there for a week I noticed that the medical providers were complaining a lot about the rooms not being stocked appropriately with supplies. A provider would come out in the middle of an office visit and become angry that there were no paper towels, no band aids, no gauze, etcetera. We all felt like we were walking on eggshells.

The office manager held a meeting and came down pretty heavy on all of us. I felt as though my job might be in jeopardy and I had only been there for a week.

I also had a lot of experience as a medical assistant, and I suggested that the MAs all get together to discuss the problem. I proposed that we come up with a checklist and place it outside the door of every treatment room. Every morning we would all be responsible to complete the checklist and stock the rooms appropriately.

This system worked and the providers were very appreciative. I was complimented by the office manager for coming up with the solution and for alleviating a constant source of stress in the practice.

Qualities: ability to handle stress, problem solver, leadership

DOS:

    ✓ Use a specific, real-life example of a stressful situation.

    ✓ State the problem.

    ✓ Describe exactly what you did to solve the problem.

    ✓ Make yourself the hero without going overboard.

DON'TS:

- ✗ Don't ramble, keep it succinct and related to the problem.
- ✗ Don't forget to make yourself the hero.
- ✗ Don't exaggerate.

**"Tell me about a time someone in your team didn't do his job and how you resolved the problem?"**

Being in a health care team requires that everyone in that team works collaboratively. If you have one employee who is having difficulty or not doing her part, it can throw off the entire team and ultimately effect patient care. Admissions committees feel that they are the gatekeepers for the PA profession, as well as their program. The committee wants to know that the applicants they select actually have leadership qualities, which means dealing with situations as they arrive.

### Example Answer

> At my last position as a supervisor, I managed several other employees, one of whom seemed to always be a step behind the rest of the team and consistently missed deadlines. I took him aside and talked with him. I discovered through the course of our discussion that he had been promoted from another department but never given the necessary training for his new position. He was terrified to ask for help because he thought that if it became known that he lacked this training he would be immediately fired. Instead, he had been struggling and essentially learning on his own.
>
> Rather than having him fired, <u>I realized what he needed was a little help.</u> We worked out a schedule where we could meet up and I could <u>mentor</u> him. By working together and helping him go over the materials and learn his job, <u>I was able to retain a valuable employee.</u> Now rather than slowing down the team, he has become an integral member.

Quality: problem solver, mentorship, leadership

DOS:

- ✓ Taking responsibility for your team members and ensuring they're all working together is a sign of a good leader.
- ✓ Motivate with praise, not with intimidation.
- ✓ Show that you have an open mind and that you can problem solve.

DON'TS:

> ✗ Don't brag about deceitful techniques you have employed in the past.
> ✗ Don't be condescending.

## "Tell me about a time when your communication skills made a difference?"

Being an effective communicator is a necessary trait to have if you are going to be a health care provider. Obviously PAs communicate with patient's every day; sometimes to explain treatment regimens or a diagnosis, and sometimes to persuade patients about why it's so important to lose weight, control their high blood pressure, or manage their diabetes. Effective communicators make better providers.

### Example Answer

> One project I worked on in college involved developing a curriculum for a program dealing with cultural similarities in everyday life. <u>The challenge was to communicate with my team members</u> and get them to be as excited about their roles in the project as I was about my role. <u>I met with them individually, drawing out any specific interests they had relative to the project.</u> I used the information from these individual sessions to assign responsibility to coincide with that interest, allowing me to bring about the best results through a team effort. The feedback from the team was positive. Everyone felt that he or she made a positive contribution in his or her own special way. It was worth the extra effort I made to listen to each individual and motivate each of them to use their strengths to develop the curriculum.

Qualities: communication, motivator

DOS:

> ✓ Communicating with a team to discuss each individual's strengths is important if you want to get the most out of their efforts.
> ✓ Show the committee that you have the ability to motivate and persuade people.

DON'TS:

> ✗ Don't talk about being aggressive.
> ✗ Don't be authoritative, be collaborative.

# Twenty-Five Behavioral Questions

1. Tell us about a time when you had to handle a stressful situation.

2. Your application states that you're a hard worker. Give us an example of a time when you worked hard.

3. Describe an interaction you've had with a patient who made an impact on you.

4. Tell us about a time when your communication skills made a difference.

5. Give us an example of a time when you took initiative.

6. You mentioned in your essay that you're good at selling new ideas to your boss and coworkers. How do you do that?

7. Have you ever been in a situation, at work or in school, where you felt it was necessary to address an ethical issue? Describe the situation.

8. Tell me about a time when you had a disagreement or confrontation with a boss or coworker.

9. If you and a colleague had a personality clash, what would you do to make it better?

10. Do you think it's important to promote team building in an organization? What steps would you take as a PA student to promote team building in the class?

11. From your perspective, describe what makes a person likeable.

12. Describe a time when you tried your hardest to accomplish something, but you still failed.

13. Talk about a time when you had to work closely with someone whose personality was very different from yours.

14. Describe a time when you struggled to build a relationship with someone important. How did you eventually overcome that?

15. We all make mistakes we wish we could take back. Tell us about a time you wish you'd handled a situation differently with a colleague.

16. Tell us about a time you were under a lot of pressure. What was going on, and how did you get through it?

17. Tell us about the first job you ever had. What did you do to learn the ropes?

18. Describe the most difficult ethical question you've had to deal with.

19. Describe a long-term project that you managed. How did you keep everything moving along in a timely manner?

20. Tell us about a time you set a goal for yourself. How did you go about ensuring that you would meet your objective?

21. Give us an example of a time you managed numerous responsibilities. How did you handle that?

22. Give us an example of a time when you had to explain something fairly complex to a frustrated client/patient/customer. How did you handle this delicate situation?

23. Tell us about your proudest professional accomplishment.

24. Tell us about a time you were dissatisfied in your work. What could have been done to make it better?

25. Tell us about a time when you worked under close supervision or extremely loose supervision. How did you handle that?

# THE MULTIPLE MINI INTERVIEW (MMI)

## What Is a MMI?

You may find that some PA programs do not use a traditional approach to the PA school interview; some use the MMI as an evaluation tool. Some PA programs recognize that the predictive value of the traditional interview on future PA school performance is low. Multiple mini interviews have been shown to be the strongest predictor of future clinical performance, professional conduct, etc.

A multiple mini interview consists of a series of short, structured interview stations used to assess noncognitive qualities, including cultural sensitivity, maturity, teamwork, empathy, reliability, and communication skills.

Prior to the start of each mini-interview rotation, candidates receive a question/scenario and have a short period of time (typically 2 to 3 minutes) to prepare an answer. (All PA programs may not use the same format for MMIs, so be open to alternative scenarios. It's possible that you may walk into the room and directly be asked questions by the interviewer.)

Upon entering the interview room, the candidate has a short exchange with the interviewer/assessor. In some cases, the interviewer observes while the action takes place between an actor and the candidate. At the end of each mini interview, the interviewer evaluates the candidate's performance while the applicant moves to the next station. This pattern is repeated through a number of stations.

Generally, the situational questions posed in a MMI touch on the following areas:

- Ethical decision making
- Critical thinking
- Communication skills
- Current health care and societal issues

Although participants must relate to the scenario posed at each station, it is important to note that the MMI is intended to test specific knowledge and the ability to think on his or her feet. As such, there are no right or wrong answers to the questions posed in a MMI, but each applicant should consider the question from a variety of perspectives.

## How Can I Prepare for a MMI?

Candidates typically exhibit anxiety in anticipation of challenging questions that may arise. Many people have difficulty formulating logical, cohesive, polished answers within the allotted preparation time prior to the start of each station.

How well you perform during the actual interview and whether you will ultimately succeed in being accepted to the program is in large measure linked to your preparation before the day of the MMI. The most effective preparation is to anticipate the questions/scenarios you will face and practice your answers.

Here are a few tips:

1. **Understand the goal:** You should aim to answer the questions in a manner that demonstrates you are capable of being an excellent student and, thereafter, an outstanding physician assistant. Make a list of the attributes that you believe are essential for success, such as integrity and the ability to think critically. Practice integrating these key attributes into your answers.

2. **Work on time management:** Many students experience difficulty with pacing and effectively answering the questions in the allotted time. Remember that once the bell has sounded, the interview must end immediately, even if you're not finished. Some PA programs may ask several questions at each station without a time limit. In this case pacing is also important. The interviewer may have several questions

prepared and you don't want to spend your allotted time answering only one or two questions. Practice 3- to 5-minute presentations in advance of your interview to get comfortable with timing. *Be sure to* wear a watch that clearly displays the time on the day of your interview; don't rely on there being a clock in the interview room. Appropriately managing your time will give you the opportunity to end the interview in an organized and effective manner.

3. **Listen carefully:** During the MMI, the interviewer will often provide prompts designed to direct you. Listen carefully to the cues provided so you can take advantage of any new information that may be introduced. The prompts may guide you to the specific issues that are the focus of each rotation.

Although success cannot be guaranteed, you can improve your performance significantly by studying the interview process, acquiring strategies to avoid common pitfalls, and knowing ways to sell yourself so that you get that seat in the class you deserve. Poise under pressure can make the difference between achieving your goals and falling just short. As you get ready for the big day, mock interviews should be a key part of your preparations. Simulating what you are about to experience will help build confidence, allowing you to remain calm and more organized on the day of your interview.

Okay, let's now take a look at some typical MMI questions that you may be asked at your PA school interview.

### "Why do you want to be a PA and not another health care professional?"

You will be asked this question in one form or another. The interviewer is looking to see if you understand the role of the PA, and exactly why you wouldn't want to be a nurse, allied health professional, nurse practitioner, or a physician.

### Example Answer

I've had several years of medical experience working with a variety of medical providers and allied health professionals. I've had the opportunity to observe the various roles of each, and I've clearly decided that I want to practice medicine as a PA. I want to be able to evaluate, diagnose, and provide a treatment plan for my patients.

As such, I ruled out becoming a nurse or allied health professional, since these health care professionals do not diagnose or prescribe treatment plans.

I've also ruled out becoming a nurse practitioner for the simple reason that I am not a nurse. To accomplish a goal of becoming a nurse practitioner, I would first have to go to nursing school, then work as a nurse for a period of time, then complete a nurse practitioner program. Given the time and financial commitment, I do not think it is feasible to pursue the NP route.

Finally, becoming a physician would be a significant investment of time and money; one that I am not able to make at this time in my life. As a PA I can fulfill my desire to practice medicine in 2 years, with less debt, and be able to start practicing relatively quickly, versus the physician route.

I welcome the dependent nature of the PA profession, and the collaborative environment that I would be working in. I'm encouraged by the consistent growth of the profession, and the fact that PA's enjoy a high satisfaction level with their patients.

After careful consideration and research of all of the above choices, I believe the PA profession is the best career choice for me.

Qualities: health care experience, maturity, critical thinking

DOS:
  ✓ Prepare for this question: either for the MMI or traditional interview.
  ✓ Consider all of the other options and tell why you've ruled them out.
  ✓ Make your answer specific to the PA profession, not health care in general.

DON'TS:
  ✗ Don't talk negatively about another profession.
  ✗ Don't say, "Because I want to help people."

## "What are three things you look for when evaluating a PA program?"

The three things I look for when evaluating a PA program include: first-time pass/fail rate on the PANCE exam, longevity of the program, and the mission of the program.

I list the first-time pass/fail rate on the PANCE as number one, because if I invest 2 or more years of my time at a PA program, as well as investing possibly over one hundred thousand dollars, I want to be sure that I will be able to pass my boards and become certified once I've completed the program. I believe the first-time pass/fail rates on the PANCE is a good indicator of a program's success. If a program does not have a high first-time pass/fail rate on the PANCE, there must be a flaw in the educational process. Although I believe that I would thoroughly prepare myself to pass the PANCE at any cost, I don't want to gamble my future on a program that does not have a proven track record of success.

The longevity of the program is also extremely important to me. Programs with longevity have had the time to refine their didactic program as well as their clinical rotation sites. I feel that if I attend a newer program, it may be a bit of a gamble. The program may be still working out the "kinks," if you will, in the didactic setting. Additionally, from my understanding, securing excellent clinical rotation sites is a bit of a trial and error proposition. It may take a few years for a program to weed out the bad rotations and replace them with better ones. I believe there is probably a direct correlation between longevity and high first-time pass/fail rates on the PANCE.

The final thing I evaluate in selecting a PA program is the mission and values of the program. I am extremely passionate about working with underserved and diverse populations. I want to attend a program that doesn't just mention "underserved areas and diversity," but actually provides clinical rotation sites in underserved areas, and possibly participates in yearly projects or events working with the underserved.

## Qualities: understanding of the PA profession and PA school

DOS:

- ✓ Prepare a list of specific things you look for in a program.
- ✓ Prepare an outline to help you create supporting material for each answer.

DON'TS:

- ✗ Don't mention geography.
- ✗ Don't mention that the program is the least expensive.

## "If you were in an auditorium and nobody knew what a PA was, how would you describe the profession?"

I would define the PA profession, talk about the history of the profession, the "dependent" nature of the profession, actual roles PAs take on in the health care system, the educational process, the future of the PA profession, and my role as a PA, and why I chose the profession.

I would explain that PAs are health care professionals licensed to practice medicine under the supervision of a licensed physician. PAs are able to evaluate, diagnose, and treat patients just like their supervising physicians. PAs prescribe medications, order and interpret lab and diagnostic studies, and formulate treatment plans. I would further explain that PAs can do approximately 80%, or more of what their physician supervisors are able to do.

I would also provide a little history about the PA profession, so the audience can get a feel for the beginnings and growth of the profession. I would explain that the first class of PA school students were educated at Duke University, and they were all former navy corpsman. Dr. Eugen Stead, the founder of the PA profession, felt that there were many former navy corpsmen who had a lot of medical experience, but had no place to enhance their skills in the civilian world.

## Quality: knowledge of the PA profession

DOS:
- ✓ Know the history of the PA profession.
- ✓ Explain why you are choosing this path.

DON'TS:
- ✗ Don't get too technical; your audience may not have any medical experience/knowledge.
- ✗ Don't just give the AAPA definition of a PA; be creative.

**"If you had to decide to give a liver transplant to a 67-year-old (female), successful member of the community, or a 22-year-old (male), active alcoholic and drug addict, whom would you choose and why?"**

This is certainly an example of an ethical question, and believe me, the interviewer doesn't want to hear you say, "As a PA I would never have to make that decision." Listen carefully to the question, provide an argument for both sides, and take a stance. Remember, there is no right or wrong answer. The interviewer wants to understand your reasoning for making your decision.

### Example Answer

First off, I would look at this liver as a precious gift that was donated by a person who recently died. I would like to think that when the donor was living and made the decision to donate his liver, he would like it to go to someone who would appreciate this gift and use it to live a longer, improved quality of life.

Having said that, I would evaluate each candidate separately, and make my decision based on facts and not emotion, or even age in this case.

At first it may seem logical to choose the 22-year-old because of his age. He would, potentially, benefit from this gift for many more years than the 67-year-old woman. However, I would also consider that he is an active alcoholic and drug addict. If he is on the transplant list and still using drugs and alcohol, I would have to consider if I truly believed he would stop using drugs and alcohol after he received the transplant.

I know that addiction is a powerful disease, and many addicts can withstand a lot of pain and still not be motivated to stop using. Some questions I would have to think about are: Would he stop using drugs and alcohol if he received the transplant? Would he be compliant with taking his daily anti-rejection medications? Would he be compliant with follow-up medical visits? Would the narcotic pain medication he would need after the surgery fuel his addiction even more?

Considering the 67-year-old female patient, I would thoroughly investigate her general health and see if she would be able to survive the surgery. If I felt she was in good enough health, besides needing the transplant, I would have to consider how long she would have to live after receiving the transplant. What if she only lived for another 5 years? What if she rejected the liver because of her age? Wouldn't the donor want the recipient to get as many years from this gift as possible?

There appears to be more questions than answers in this case. However, I think the decision would be an easy one for me. I would choose the 67-year-old female over the 22-year-old active alcoholic and drug addict.

I believe if the young male patient is on a liver transplant list, yet still abusing alcohol and drugs, he is not likely to stop using alcohol and drugs just because he receives a new liver. In fact, he may look at the new liver as a reason to keep using drugs and alcohol because he now has a new lease on life, if you will. I feel it is unlikely he would be compliant with his anti-rejection medication regimen, his addiction would be fueled even more by the narcotic pain medication he would receive after the surgery, and considering these circumstances, this gift may only last for 6 months, or even less.

I believe that if the 22-year-old had been clean and sober for a year, I may have to think differently about his situation. But from the knowledge I have right now, I would not give him the benefit of the doubt.

On the other hand, the 67-year-old female is much more likely to take care of this gift. She is likely to take her anti-rejection medication, keep her follow-up appointments, and live a clean lifestyle. She could possibly live another 20 years with this transplant. In my mind I believe 20 years, or even 10 years, beats 6 months.

In summary, the age factor would not come into play, it is the health and lifestyle of the recipient that I would base my decision on. Given these criteria, I believe the 67-year-old woman is the best fit.

Qualities: judgment, decisive, problem solver, critical thinking

DOS:
- ✓ Look at the big picture.
- ✓ Consider the positives and negatives in making your decision.
- ✓ Make a decision based on facts and not emotion.

DON'TS:
- ✗ Don't make a superficial decision based on the age of the patients.
- ✗ Don't be afraid to play devil's advocate.
- ✗ Don't be judgmental.

**"You are a PA working in an inner-city family practice clinic. You have a husband and wife on your schedule today coming in for HIV test results. You know ahead of time that the husband tested positive and the wife tested negative. You call the husband into the room first, and advise him that he tested positive for HIV. The first words out of his mouth are, *Don't tell my wife!* How would you handle this situation?"**

HIV is frequently an interview topic in one form or another. It is important to research the medical laws relating to HIV reporting in the state where the program is located, before your interview. It is also important to discuss the facts, and not be judgmental or emotional.

### Example Answer

As I am not currently a PA, and therefore I do not know for sure what the law and regulations are with respect to HIV reporting and disclosure in each state, I can only provide the answer to this situation based on the knowledge and information I have for HIV testing and privacy here in Connecticut.

In Connecticut, medical law permits the medical provider, under certain circumstances, to inform or warn partners that they may have been exposed to HIV if: there is a significant belief of risk of transmission to that partner, if the provider has reason to believe the HIV positive patient will not disclose his HIV status to his partner or spouse, and if the provider discloses the fact that he intends to disclose the information.

Before discussing my intent to notify his wife of a potential HIV exposure, I would: educate the patient about how to cope with the emotional consequences of learning his HIV status, inform him about potential discrimination issues, discuss behavior modification issues to prevent transmission, inform the patient about medical treatments available and services and support centers available, and discuss the need to notify partners.

After going over this information, I would approach the patient about revealing his HIV status to his wife. If the patient still asks me not to tell his wife, I would advise him that although I could not reveal his HIV status to his wife directly, I can, and will, inform her that she may have been exposed to HIV. However, I always believe it is better to converse with a patient directly before taking the next step.

As a medical provider, I believe I would be obligated to go one step further in trying to convince my patient that he should speak to his wife about his HIV status. I would reason with him that when I notify his wife of a possible HIV exposure, she will probably "put two and two" together and realize it was him who has HIV because this is the reason you both came to this office visit. I would offer to have he and his wife meet with our professional HIV counselor, who deals with these situations every day.

If the patient still refuses to allow me to notify his wife of his HIV status, I would talk to him about the treatment options available, the importance of using protection when having sex, and the possible legal consequences that may be involved if he knowingly infects another person.

I would then meet with his wife, provide her with her test results, and advise her that she may have been exposed to HIV. I would offer her the same counseling I offered to her husband. After doing so, I would feel comfortable that I followed all of the medical-legal issues, and know that I did my best to work with the husband to notify his wife about his HIV status. Beyond that, there is nothing else that I could do.

Qualities: knowledgeable, reasoning, decision making, communication skills

Multiplier: knowing the specific laws relating to HIV reporting in the state where you are interviewing

DOS:
- ✓ Research HIV laws for every state you have an interview.
- ✓ Answer the question in a methodical, rationale manner.
- ✓ Ultimately, decide to do the right thing no matter what.

DON'TS:
- ✗ Don't forget to do your homework.
- ✗ Don't be judgmental.
- ✗ Don't force the patient to tell his wife, use your communication skills and reasoning to persuade him.
- ✗ Don't violate HIPPA laws

# Fifteen Multiple Mini Interview Questions

1. Joe is a pizza-delivery worker. The pizza shop he works for guarantees to deliver the pizza within 30 minutes, or else the customer does not have to pay. On Joe's most recent delivery, he spots a woman bleeding on the street. There is no one else around, and the woman seems unable to move by herself. However, Joe knows that if he returns empty-handed again, he will be fired from this job, which he most desperately needs. What do you think Joe should do? Justify your solution in terms of practical and ethical considerations.

2. If you walked out of your house one morning and found a shoebox with $100,000 dollars inside, and your name was printed on the top, what would you do with the money?

3. Why do you want to be a PA and not another health care professional?

4. What are three things you look for when evaluating a program?

5. What would you do if you don't get accepted this year?

6. Tell me about the last PA you shadowed.

7. Tell me about your health care experiences.

8. If you could strengthen your application, what would it be and why?

9. If you were in an auditorium and nobody knew what a PA was, how would you describe the profession?

10. What is interdisciplinary medicine and how is it helping the quality of patient care?

11. How do you see yourself helping in underserved communities?

12. What does managed care mean to you?

13. Are you a fan of the Affordable Care Act? Why or why not?

14. If you had to make the final decision on whether to change the PA profession's name from *physician assistant* to *physician associate,* which would you choose and why?

15. You friend confides in you that his mother was recently diagnosed with breast cancer. He tells you that he really feels he should be there for her and he plans to drop out of school. How would you council him?

# ETHICAL INTERVIEW QUESTIONS

Having high ethical standards is a must for anyone who works in the health care profession. As PAs we face ethical challenges every day. We cannot afford to make decisions based on emotion; rather we have to make decisions based on the right thing to do.

You will be asked ethical questions at your interview. You will be given hypothetical scenarios to evaluate, and you will be expected to choose an answer, along with your justification for your choice.

You cannot study for ethical questions and you are not expected to know what it's like to be a PA. However, I will present a few scenarios here to give you an idea what to expect at your interview. There are also many more ethical scenarios, with answers, presented in my book, *How to Ace the Physician Assistant School Interview.*

## Sample Ethical Questions

**"Do you believe all individuals have a right to health care in this country?"**

### Example Answer

> I believe that all people in this country should have access to health care. I also believe that my job as a medical provider would be to provide the highest quality health care for any patient that presents to me for treatment, regardless of her ability to pay.
>
> As far as patients having a "right" to healthcare, I believe that is a political decision made by legislators, and not medical providers.

Qualities: reasoning, nonjudgmental

DOS:

- ✓ Think the situation through, and realize the limitations of the health care provider.
- ✓ Mention that health care providers have an obligation to treat all patients who present to them for care.

DON'TS:

- ✗ Don't get into a political discussion.
- ✗ Don't be authoritative, be collaborative.

## "Tell me about a time when you had to handle an ethical dilemma?"

### Example Answer

During a biochemistry examination, I saw one of my classmates using a "cheat sheet" to answer the questions.

I always think it is best to confront a person directly if I have a concern about any type of discrepancy. I approached my classmate after class and said to him; "I feel like you may have been cheating during this exam, am I correct?" he admitted to me that he was cheating and told me that he had a lapse in judgment. He confided in me that he had a difficult time understanding the material, and he was afraid to ask for help. I realized that I had two options: report him to the professor, or offer to help him study for future exams if he needed the help.

I decided to offer him help with the material, and he was very appreciative. I also advised him that if I caught him cheating again, I would have no choice but to report him to the professor.

As it turned out, he accepted my help and did very well for the rest of the semester.

I am the type of person who believes that everyone has lapses of judgment at one time or another, and I believe in giving second chances when appropriate.

Qualites: compassion, being a real person

DOS:
   ✓ Confront the student before going to the professor.
   ✓ Be real.
   ✓ Act with integrity and honesty.

DON'TS:
   ✗ Compromise your own ethics.
   ✗ Ignore the situation.
   ✗ Don't accuse the student.
   ✗ Don't tell the committee what you think they want to hear.

## "What would you do if you knew your supervising physician was committing Medicare fraud by overbilling for his services?"

### Example Answer

> I would first ask to speak to my supervising physician in private. I would tell him that I feel he is overbilling Medicare patients, and that I am very uncomfortable participating in a practice which uses unethical billing practices. I would advise the physician that ethics is extremely important to me, and if he continued to bill Medicare inappropriately, I would leave the practice and would consider reporting his actions to Medicare.

Qualities: integrity, honesty

DOS:
- ✓ Be true to yourself.
- ✓ Confront your supervisor, first, before taking any other actions.
- ✓ Advise your supervisor of the consequences of his actions and what action you will take if he does not change his unethical practices.

DON'TS:
- ✗ Don't be afraid to confront anyone acting unethically.
- ✗ Don't put yourself at risk by ignoring the problem.
- ✗ Don't be aggressive when speaking about the dilemma.

# Fifteen Ethical Questions

1. What do you believe compromises the ethical workplace?
2. Have you worked for a company that had a code of conduct, and did you have positive or negative experiences there?
3. Have you taken a course or had any training in medical ethics?
4. How does being an ethical individual differ from being an ethical corporation?
5. Would you ever lie for us?
6. Tell us about a time that you were challenged ethically.
7. When you've had ethical issues arise at work, whom did you consult?
8. I see you've worked with people from different cultures. What ethics and values did you find you had in common, and where did you differ?
9. Do you believe that all individuals have a right to health care in this country?

10. What would you do if you witnessed a classmate cheating on a test?

11. What would you do if your supervising physician asked you to write an order for a medication you thought might harm your patient, what would you do?

12. What if a nurse refused to carry out one of your orders?

13. What would you do if you ordered a medication for a patient in the hospital, and you realized after it was given to that patient, that you prescribed the wrong medication.

14. What would you do if you walked on the floor one day, and one of the nurses tells you that she saw your friend, and colleague of 10 years, take controlled medications out of the narcotics locker and put them in his pocket?

15. What would you do if you noticed your supervising physician billing at a higher level for those patients on Medicaid, and when you confronted him about it, he tells you that since Medicaid does not reimburse well, he needs to bill at the higher level to make up for lost revenue.

## SITUATIONAL INTERVIEW QUESTIONS

Responses to situational questions can make or break an interview. An interviewer uses situational interviewing techniques to elicit specific examples of an applicant's ability to perform under stress, work as a team player, and communicate with colleagues. Additionally, the interviewer will want to know how well you understand the role of a PA.

**"A coworker tells you in confidence that she plans to call in sick while actually taking a week's vacation. What would you do and why?"**

### Example Answer

I would tell this coworker that being dishonest to her boss, as well as her coworkers, is not wise, and being dishonest in her job is wrong. I would explain how we all want more vacation time, but we have to earn it—and that taking this extra time hurts everyone in the department because the person's absence will affect productivity.

Qualities: assertiveness, team player

DOS:

✓ Be assertive, not aggressive.

✓ Point out the situation for a team perspective.

DON'TS:

✗ Don't ignore the situation.

✗ Don't be condescending.

**"What would you do if the work of a subordinate or team member was not up to expectations?"**

### Example Answer

> Luckily, I have quite a bit of previous team experience, and have faced this situation a few times in the past—so let me tell you how I've learned to handle the issue. The important first step in dealing with an underperforming subordinate or team member is honest communication—talking with the person can lead to some surprising discoveries, such as the person not understanding the assigned tasks or being overwhelmed with the assignment. Once I discovered the problem, I could then forge a solution that usually solved the problem and allowed the work to move forward. So often in situations like this, the problem is some combination of miscommunications and unrealistic expectations.

Qualities: team player, communicator, problem solver, experienced

DOS:

✓ Communicate directly with the employee.

✓ Be honest.

✓ Consider the problem from both sides.

DON'TS:

✗ Don't go directly to the supervisor without talking to the employee first.

✗ Don't assume your subordinate is purposely underperforming.

**"How would you deal with a colleague at work with whom you seem to be unable to build a successful working relationship?"**

**Example Answer**

This situation would certainly be unique to me. Ever since I can remember, I've had a knack for finding something in everyone that then becomes common ground for a friendship and/or good working relationship. Certainly there are all types of people, some less motivated to work in teams or unhappy in their jobs, but we're all people when you strip away titles and such—and it's at that base level in which I find a connection which results in some degree of rapport—even when few others can do so. For example, in my senior year of college, I was placed onto a team that had one member that the rest of the team disliked. The team member was kind of an outcast, but I knew we needed this full commitment to make this project work. Even though I was not the team leader, I took it upon myself to forge a connection—and discovered we had a mutual passion for horses. We did not become best friends, but through our common interest, I was able to build enough rapport to connect and engage him as a key team member. There is always something that bonds us all together—it's just harder to find with some people than with others.

Qualities: cooperative, leadership, team oriented, communication skills

DOS:
- ✓ Try to find common ground with the person.
- ✓ Have a positive attitude.
- ✓ Be cooperative.
- ✓ Take the high ground.

DON'TS:
- ✗ Don't ignore the situation.
- ✗ Don't get a resentment toward your colleague.
- ✗ Don't forget the goal is teamwork.

# Fifteen Sample Situational Questions

1. In health care, we deal with all types of patients and coworkers. Explain how you have dealt with a difficult person at work. How did you handle it? What were the results?

2. What would you do if you ordered a medication for a patient, but the nurse refused to carry it out?

3. What would you do if you worked in the emergency room and wanted to admit a very sick, 9 year-old, but the attending physician wanted to send her home?

4. What is the biggest challenge you've faced, and how did you solve it?

5. Describe a time when you had to defend an unpopular decision you made.

6. Describe a recent situation where you dealt with an upset coworker or customer.

7. Tell us about your most difficult boss and how you were able to deal with him or her.

8. What would you do if you were working on an important project and all of a sudden the priorities were changed?

9. Please describe a time when your work was criticized by your boss or other coworkers.

10. Share with us a time you went the extra mile to resolve a problem or accomplish something.

11. Team members you've been assigned to lead during a new project object to your vision and ideas for implementation. What specifically would you do to address their objections?

12. You're responsible for an important project near completion but receive another important project that must be completed immediately. How do you multitask and prioritize?

13. When a subordinate is performing below average, what specific steps do you take to correct the problem?

14. You're responsible for ensuring a large amount of work to be finished before a school project is due. A classmate decides to use sick time to take an entire week off from school. What would you do to address the problem?

15. What would you do if you knew your supervising physician was absolutely wrong about an important work-related issue?

## ILLEGAL INTERVIEW QUESTIONS

Similar to writing good test questions, selecting appropriate interview questions is a skill. Many PA school admissions committee members are not professional interviewers and may not even know the rules about illegal interview questions. PA school interview questions should be directed at your qualifications to become a PA, and not about your personal information.

When dealing with illegal interview questions, ask yourself: "Do I want to be right, or do I want to be effective?" In other words, if you are asked a question that you know is illegal to ask, you may not want to say, "Hey, that's an illegal question." I suggest you assume the interviewer is asking the illegal question out of ignorance and not to trip you up.

For the purposes of this chapter, we'll assume the interviewer is ignorant to the rules about asking illegal questions, and I'll show you how to answer the (underlying) question, without having to expose any personal information.

What questions are illegal?

- Questions about marital status/family status
- Questions about age
- Personal questions
- Questions about disabilities
- Questions about your arrest record
- Questions about military service
- Questions about politics/affiliations
- Questions about race, color, or religion

Here are some examples of typical illegal questions and answers.

### "Do you have any children?"

(The interviewer may ask you this question to determine in his mind ("fortune telling") if you will need to take the time off from school or rotations to stay home with your children.)

#### Example Answer

> There is absolutely no reason why I will not be able to show up for class or clinical rotations every day.

Notice the applicant recognizes this as an illegal question and answers the real question being asked, "Are you going to be missing a lot of time because you don't have day care?"

**"How old are you?"**

(This question probably has more to do with maturity than chronological age.)

> I've accomplished all of the academic prerequisites and health care experience requirements to qualify for this program. I know what it takes to become a good physician assistant, and I am ready to embrace the challenges of PA school.

**"How much do you weigh?"**

(This is a rude and illegal question to say the least. The interviewer may be thinking you cannot handle the job if you are overweight or obese. The interviewer may also be extremely judgmental.)

> Weight has never been an issue for me. I've never had a problem performing any of my job duties.

**"I see you're not moving your left arm, did you hurt yourself?"**

(This is a "fishing" question to see if you have a disability that would interfere with your duties as a PA.)

> I'm fine, thank you.

**You have an interesting accent; which country are you from?**

(Inquiries about a person's citizenship or country of birth are unlawful and imply discrimination on the basis of national origin.)

> That's an interesting question. Is this information pertinent to my application?

**"Have you ever been arrested?"**

(Upon completion of PA school, you will have to undergo a background check to see if you qualify for a medical license. If you have any felonies or drug convictions, you will be disqualified. You may want to check this out for yourself before applying to PA school. However, if you have been arrested for any minor offenses but not convicted, you don't have to divulge that information. If you have a current arrest, the admissions committee can ask you about that and take it into consideration when making a decision about your candidacy.)

| No, I've never been convicted of a criminal offense. |

## "Are you a Republican or a Democrat?"

(This is a loaded question. Never talk about politics at an interview, unless you want to sabotage your chances of being accepted.)

| It's my policy never to discuss politics with anyone. |

## "What is your religion?"

(All religious questions are illegal. Interviewers may ask about your religious background to see if you will have any conflict working Saturdays or Sundays.)

| My religious preference is very personal. |

# Twenty Sample Illegal Questions

1. Are you Caucasian/African American/Hispanic?
2. Do you attend church/synagogue/mosque?
3. Are you married?
4. Are you planning to have children?
5. Are you pregnant?
6. Who is going to watch your children when you are in school?
7. When were you born?
8. When is your birthday?
9. How tall are you?
10. What is your sexual orientation?
11. What medications do you take?
12. Do you have any mental health issues?
13. Do you have heart disease?
14. Have you ever been treated for alcoholism or drug addiction?
15. Do you have an eating disorder?
16. Will you need us to make any accommodations in order for you to complete the program?
17. Where were you born?
18. Are you a citizen?
19. Your last name sounds Italian, is it?
20. Who did you vote for in the last election?

# HYPOTHETICAL QUESTIONS: IF YOU WERE AN ANIMAL/COLOR/FRUIT/TREE, WHAT WOULD IT BE?

It is becoming increasingly common for interviewers to throw in some unusual questions during interviews rather than sticking to the tried and true. This could be for a number of reasons: they want to see if you can think on your feet, think creatively, say something illuminating about yourself, and possibly demonstrate a sense of humor.

The following hypothetical questions may seem a bit odd, or even a bit ridiculous. You may be asking yourself:

- "What difference does it make what color I would be?"
- "Is this a psychiatric interview, or an interview for PA school?"
- "If I say an apple versus an orange, will that answer affect my score?"

How ridiculous, right? Well, you may think these hypothetical questions are ridiculous, but the fact of the matter is that programs frequently ask the following hypothetical questions and the perfect applicant knows how to provide a smart answer.

Let's look at some of the most common hypothetical questions and answers.

**"If you were an animal, what would it be?"**

> If I were an animal, I would be an eagle. An eagle is a bird that can soar ten thousand feet above the ground and see for three square miles. At the same time, an eagle can also see the tiniest mouse crawling on the ground on the desert floor.

The implication is that you have the ability to see the "big picture," while also being able to focusing on the smallest details.

**"If you were a color, what would it be?"**

> If I were a color, I would be charcoal gray. Charcoal gray is an uncommon color that represents maturity, leadership, and it blends well with any other color.

By choosing charcoal gray as your color, you are telling the committee that you are an individual, not a carbon-copy applicant. You are also saying that you are mature, and that you're a team player.

Are you starting to see the point? You should choose your answers to coincide with some of the qualities of the perfect applicant.

Let's try another.

## "If you were a fruit, what would it be?"

I would be a banana. A banana has substance and blends well in a fruit salad.

You are telling the committee that you are a strong applicant and that you would be a good classmate (team player).

## "If you were a tree, what would it be?"

If I were a tree, I would be a palm tree. In a severe storm, a palm tree can sway all the way to the ground without breaking, yet it always bounces right back up once the storm is over.

The qualities are flexibility and resilience.

There are no right or wrong answers to hypothetical questions. You job is to think on your feet and come up with an answer that matches the qualities you possess, and the qualities the admissions committee is looking for in the perfect applicant.

# SUMMARY

We covered a lot of ground in this chapter. I hope you now appreciate how much *work* it takes to become the perfect applicant. You learned about the tailoring method, and how to find the qualities each program looks for in future students. You also learned about using multipliers to supercharge your answers. By infusing qualities and multipliers into the answers you provide at the PA school interview, you will blow away the competition.

But not so fast! Effectively building trust and credibility with the admissions committee involves more than just providing great answers to the interview questions. Answering the questions is only the *verbal* component of your message, and the spoken message has three components: the verbal, vocal, and the visual. And believe it or not, the visual and vocal components can weigh much more than the verbal component. Confused? Let's take a look at the next chapter to see exactly what I mean.

# [CHAPTER 8]

# The Interview
# (Part Two)

## INTRODUCTION

Now that you've learned the tailoring method to infuse qualities and multipliers into the PA school interview answers, it's time to look at another very important aspect of the PA school interview process. In addition to answering questions, the admissions committee also wants to learn more about you as a person. For instance:

- Are you likable?
- Are you a compassionate person?
- Do you fully understand the role of a PA?
- Are you mature?
- Can you handle stress?
- Can the interviewer(s) visualize you as a colleague?
- Are you overconfident, or have a sense of entitlement?
- Are you trustworthy?
- Are you energetic?
- Are you an effective communicator?
- Would the interviewer want you taking care of his/her mother?

## High-Impact Communication

To claim your seat in next year's class, you will need to develop certain skills and behaviors that will enhance your position with the interview committee. The first of these behaviors is charisma, or having extraordinary personal power or charm. To some, charisma comes natural, but more often than not it must be learned. Charisma is the result of a series of behaviors through which someone has a powerful and positive impact on others. This is exactly what you want to accomplish at your interview; use charisma to build the bridge to credibility and trust.

As a prior admissions committee member, I've interviewed many applicants who simply could not make that personal connection at the interview. These applicants obviously looked great on paper, or they wouldn't have made it to the interview phase. However, these applicants could not move beyond facts, figures, and jargon to make a connection. In contrast, the applicants who scored highest at the interview knew how to communicate effectively and persuasively, and above all, they were absolutely believable. They understood how to project openness, enthusiasm, and energy. The ability to communicate effectively is the single most important skill you need to succeed as a PA. I think we've all had an experience with a medical provider who was very dry and impersonal. She may have graduated from Harvard, but if you don't connect with her at a personal level, you may not return for another visit.

Communication is a contact sport. As I mentioned already, looking good on paper will only get you so far. If you are unable to make an emotional connection with your audience, you're likely to be rejected. I witnessed this phenomenon over and over again. In contrast, I interviewed many applicants who looked average on paper, but they made such an emotional impact at the interview I scored them higher than I had anticipated on the basis of their application alone. Creating an emotional connection with your interviewer(s) is crucial to your success.

## Creating Emotional Impact

You must learn to *sell* yourself to create emotional impact. You may be thinking "sell myself?" I'm not a salesperson. Really? Don't you have to sell your ideas to people on a daily basis? I know that I have to sell my children on why it's important to do their homework and perform well in school. I sell my patients on why it's important to take their cholesterol medication or risk getting heart disease. I sell my obese patients on why it's important to lose weight if they want to live a long, healthy life. Finally, and most importantly, I have to sell my wife on why I want to spend a lot of money on a new toy! We're *all* selling something!

What are you selling? Have you thought about it? I know many of you are uncomfortable with the word selling. However, you will have to sell yourself to the admissions committee at your interview. You will have to give them a good reason why you, among all of the competition, deserve a seat in the upcoming class. Using the tailoring method, introduced in the previous chapter, to answer the interview questions is a good start. But as you'll see, providing exceptional answers to the interview questions is only a small piece of the puzzle.

## The Secret

If you understand that you need to sell yourself to the admissions committee, then make sure you also understand this critical point: *The admissions committee selects candidates on the basis of emotion (likability, credibility, and trust) and justifies that decision with the facts (GPA, GRE scores, medical experience).* If you understand this simple secret, you will understand why you cannot rely on your CASPA application alone at your interview, nor you can rely on the answers you provide to the interview questions to be offered a seat in the upcoming class. You must make an emotional connection with the committee members to seal the deal.

For example, applicant #1 and applicant #2 come to the interview with the *exact* same GPA, GRE scores, medical experience, and volunteer hours. During the course of applicant #1's interview, his answers to the interview questions are spot on. However, he fails to make eye contact, he is not wearing a suit, he rarely smiles, and he speaks in a monotone voice. Applicant #2 comes in wearing a clean and well-pressed suit, she has a big, genuine smile on her face, she looks everyone in the eye when answering the questions, and she has great intonation and inflection in her voice. She is also spot on with her answers to the interview questions.

After these applicants leave the interview room, the committee does not take out a piece of paper and compare the facts: grades, test scores, answers to interview questions, etc. They make their decision based on emotion and justify the decision with the facts. When applicant #1 leaves the room, the committee member(s) might say, "I didn't like him, and I'm not crazy about his medical experience." When applicant #2 leaves the room, they might say, "Wow, I really like her, and she has excellent medical experience, a great GPA, and great GRE scores." Applicant #2 is going to score much higher than applicant #1.

Yes, on paper both applicants are identical. However, applicant #2 used high-impact communication skills to make that emotional connection and score higher than applicant #1 with the same credentials. And notice how they justify their decision: "…and she has excellent medical experience, a great GPA, and great GRE scores." Remember, they both have identical stats on paper!

In my 3 years on Yale's admissions committee, all of the decisions were made the same way. "I like her," "I don't like him." Connecting with the emotional center of the interviewer's brain is the key to success!

## Three Key Points to Remember

Creating emotional impact is crucial to your success as a PA school applicant. Personal impact is a powerful way to achieve whatever you want in your personal life and career. Consider these three key points before interviewing:

1. **The spoken word is almost the exact opposite of the written word**

   The written word is a one-dimensional medium for communicating facts and transferring information. The spoken word, however, is multidimensional and includes a kaleidoscope of nonverbal cues such as posture, eye contact, energy, volume, intonation, and much more. If you want to make an emotional impact, and motivate and persuade the admissions committee, you must master the spoken word and learn to make such nonverbal cues work for you rather than against you.

2. **What you say must be believed for it to have impact**

   If the committee senses that you are less than forthright with even one interview question, you will build a wall of distrust that you probably will not be able to overcome. For your message to be believed, *you* must be believed.

   I once interviewed a woman who applied to Yale's program, and she was in a group interview with myself and two other female admissions committee members. She was a nontraditional applicant; an accomplished, Off-Broadway actress. She presented us with a very fancy and off-beat résumé (which we didn't ask for, by the way). Located on the bottom right-hand corner of the résumé, below all of her Off-Broadway credits, she wrote, "Special Talents: I can tie a cherry stem into a knot with my tongue." Although this particular talent may be relevant to her role as an actress, it was completely inappropriate for a PA school application, and she had already lost her credibility with me and my fellow interviewers before she stepped foot into the interview room.

One of my colleagues who wasn't too pleased with that note on her résumé asked the applicant to comment on her "most memorable patient." The applicant started to cry and talk about her mother's diagnosis of cancer. After the applicant explained that her mother had been in remission for several years, my colleague asked her point blank, "How do we know you're not acting now?" Ouch! The candidate became very silent, stopped crying, and she knew the interview was over at that point. She lost her credibility before she even stepped into the room.

A person's gut feeling as to whether they like and believe someone is usually based on emotion, not logic. If your voice cracks, or your hands are fidgety, or you cannot make solid eye contact, you'll probably lose credibility with your audience.

### 3. Believability is determined at the subconscious level

Perhaps this is the most important point to remember. How do we determine whether we believe someone? Can you build believability out of a mountain of facts and figures? Absolutely not. You cannot even build trust out of a stack of eloquently crafted words. Authoritative credentials, a title, or a letter of recommendation from a "big shot" may give you a little credibility and get you to the interview, but you still have to be believable to close the sale.

How do you make yourself more believable? First, you must make eye contact. Without good eye contact the committee members may become suspicious of you and wonder what you are hiding. Be sure to smile. Don't become so self-involved and nervous that you forget to relax and smile. Smiling is infectious and will help you and the committee members relax. Also, use open gestures. Don't sit at the table with your arms folded tightly over your chest. Keep your arms and hands open, which will support the fact that you are an open-minded person. Use a firm handshake. There is nothing worse than a wet, sweaty handshake. Finally, have good posture and project a strong voice.

# Interviewers are Bombarded with Visual Stimuli that Register at the Preconscious Level

From the moment we walk into the interview, we begin giving off a series of verbal and nonverbal cues. Do you walk into a room tall, or do you slump? Do you have a firm handshake? Do you refer to your patients as "legs" and "arms," or do you refer to them by name? Do you refer to nurses in a derogatory manner, or do you give them the respect they deserve as colleagues?

An enormous amount of communication is taking place as thousands of multichannel impressions are carried to the brain. Most impressions register at the preconscious level. As a result of the impressions, the brain forms a continuous stream of emotional judgments and assessments: Do I trust this person? Is she honest, evasive, threatening, or friendly? Is he interesting, boring, warm, cold, or anxious? Is she confident, insecure, or perhaps hiding something?

The emotional judgment that forms in your preconscious mind about the speaker determines whether you will tune in or tune out his or her message. If you distrust someone at the emotional level, little of what that person says will get through.

# Getting to Trust

How do we use our natural self to reach the emotional center of our listeners? **You've got to be believed to be heard.** When dealing with the admissions committee, trust and believability are synonymous. You can't have one without the other. To communicate effectively with the committee, they must trust you. And to win their trust, you must be believable. Belief occurs at the gut level; it's acceptance on faith, it's emotionally based, and it bypasses the intellect.

During the interview, each committee member sifts through your nuances of behavior. Does your voice quiver, or does it project authority? Do your eyes flicker hesitantly or gaze unflinchingly? Is your posture confident or diffident? These nuances of behavior speak the language of trust.

People learn as babies who they trust and why. One day my son Eddie and I were at the airport on our way to Orlando, Florida, where I was to present a seminar. While sitting in the chairs by our gate, a toddler playfully strolled over to us with a smile on her face from ear to ear. She was cooing and drooling and having a grand old time. Eddie and I played peekaboo with her, causing her to shriek with laughter and excitement. Then she suddenly strolled over to a man sitting next to us and smiled playfully at him. Without saying a word, he gave her a look that said, "I'm not interested in you little girl. Go away!" The little girl's face went from a huge smile to a little pout. She ran from the man and knew that he represented trouble; he wasn't safe.

You cannot communicate with a baby using words. Instead, infants relate to facial expressions, energy, and sound. A baby responds with the same set of verbal cues. The smile is the language of our emotional centers. Even a baby knows that a person who doesn't smile lacks warmth and safety. We learn early in life that the people we should trust are those who (genuinely) smile. To communicate effectively, we must relearn the language of trust.

Did you ever meet someone and instantly like or dislike that person but not know why? When you meet someone for the first time, the emotional center in your brain receives thousands of nonverbal cues that are registered at the preconscious level. Your intuition comes from this; you form an almost-immediate impression of that person. You form an impression that is detailed and often richly colored with emotion.

Most candidates approach the interview as though their essay, grades, and GRE scores are what count most. They fail to realize that when they leave that interview, the individual committee members don't comment on logic and reason. Rather, they typically say, "I like her," or "I don't believe him," or "There's something about her that I really like."

Some people can naturally do this without understanding how it works. The candidate who knows how to speak the language of the brain's emotional center—the language of trust—is the candidate most likely to be believed and accepted. That language communicates very rapidly and effectively.

## The Likability Factor

In 1984, President Reagan ran for reelection against Walter Mondale (most of you probably weren't even born then). A Gallup Poll examined three areas with respect to each candidate: (1) issues, (2) party affiliation, and (3) likability. On the issues, the candidates were considered dead even. The Democrat clearly had the edge when it came to party affiliation. With respect to likability, however, Reagan had the edge and won the election. It was the personality factor that dominated.

As applicants, we pride ourselves on having a great grade point average, test scores, and years of hands-on medical experience. But when it's time to interview, it's your likability that determines whether you receive a letter of acceptance or a letter of rejection. As soon as you walk into that interview room, it's the visual connection that sets the beginning of trust and believability.

## The Eye Factor

The eye is the only sensory organ that contains brain cells. Memory experts invariably link the objects they remember to a visual image. Research shows that it's the visual image that makes the greatest impact in communication.

In the 1960s, Professor Albert Mehrabian pioneered the understanding of the effectiveness of the spoken message. He looked at three factors relating to the spoken message:

- The *verbal* message, or the actual words that we use, are what most applicants concentrate on, but this is actually the most insignificant part of the spoken message.
- The *vocal* component is made up of the intonation, projection, and resonance of your spoken message.
- The *visual* message. **It is the visual message, however, the emotion and expression of your body and face as you speak, that carries the most weight.**

Professor Mehrabian also found that the degree of consistency or inconsistency among those three elements determines the believability of your message. The more the three factors harmonize, the more believable you are as a candidate. If your verbal message is not in harmony with your body language, you send a mixed signal to the emotional center of the other person's brain. Your message may or may not get through to the decision-making, rational portion of your brain. Mehrabian quantified the three components of the spoken message as follows:

- The verbal component = 7%
- The vocal component = 38%
- The visual component = 55%

In other words, what you see is what you get. If you come into the interview room yawning or dressed inappropriately, nothing you do or say will help you. The interviewer is likely to shut you out immediately and not hear a word you have to say.

# HOW DO YOU ENHANCE YOUR MESSAGE?

## Eye Contact

The first way to enhance your communication is with eye contact. This is the number-one skill you should develop before you interview. Three rules and exercises for maintaining eye contact follow:

### Rules

1. Use involvement rather than intimacy or intimidation.
2. Count to 5 (involvement), then look away; if you are in an interview with three committee members, be sure to make eye contact with all three while answering the question. Use the 5-second rule above.
3. Don't dart your eyes; this represents a lack of confidence.

### Exercises

1. **Use video feedback.** Tape yourself speaking with someone and watch for your use or violation of the three rules.
2. **Practice one-on-one.** Have a conversation with someone you trust and ask that person for direct feedback with respect to the rules.
3. **Practice with a paper audience.** Draw smiley faces on sticky notes and then place them on a chair and practice making eye contact, counting to 5, and looking away.

## Posture and Movement

The next way to enhance your message is with posture and movement. A good posture commands attention, and movement shows confidence. Walk into the room standing tall. Don't slump. When you speak to your interviewer, don't be afraid to add movement to your message. You don't have to wave your hands all over the room, but use open gestures to come across as a friendly, open-minded person. Four rules for posture are:

### Rules

1. Stand tall.
2. Watch your lower body; don't lean back on one hip or rock back and forth.
3. Get in the ready position; lean slightly forward if you're sitting, or on the balls of your feet if you're standing.
4. Use movement to show that you're excited, enthusiastic, and confident.

**Exercises**

1. Walk away from the wall.

   Stand with your back against a wall, heels pressed against the wall along with your head, neck, and shoulders. Try to push the small of your back into the wall. Now simply walk away from the wall and feel how upright and correct your posture becomes. Try to shake off this posture; you can't. Practice this exercise daily so that when you walk into the interview room, you'll command attention.

2. Use the ready position.

   Remember, if you're standing, sit up slightly on the balls of your feet. If you are sitting, lean slightly forward toward the interviewer.

## Dress and Appearance

The third way to enhance your message is with dress and appearance. You get only 2 seconds to make your initial impression on your interviewers. If you blow it, it may take more than 30 minutes to recover, and most interviews last for only 20 minutes. So, it is critical to make a good first impression.

When you dress up for an interview, only 10% of your skin should show. Be sure that your face is well shaven or your makeup is not too overbearing. Comb or style your hair, avoid wearing extravagant jewelry, clean and trim your nails, and use cologne or perfume sparingly.

**Rules**

1. Be appropriate—when in Rome . . .

2. Be conservative; when in doubt, dress up.

3. Men, always button your jacket.

4. Use perfume and cologne sparingly.

5. Always bring a small mirror and check your face and teeth before interviewing.

**Exercises**

1. Get feedback. Ask friends and relatives to assess how well you present yourself. Be open to constructive criticism.

2. Be observant; read fashion magazines. Find a style with which you are comfortable. Don't go over the edge, however.

## Gestures and Smile

The final way to enhance your message is with gestures and your smile. Do you speak with conviction, enthusiasm, and passion? Are you friendly or stuffy? Do you speak with open gestures and a warm smile, or are you a fig-leaf flasher, always covering and uncovering your groin with your hands? (a common nervous tick). Remember, openness equals likability. Here are three rules for gestures and smiling:

### Rules

1. Be aware of nervous gestures and stop them.
2. Lift the apples of your cheeks—smile. Make believe that you have apples on your cheekbones and try to lift them up to your forehead.
3. Feel your smile, but beware: phony smiles don't work.

### Exercises

1. Imitate someone whom you feel is an effective communicator and play the part with gusto. Get used to using open gestures and expressions.
2. Be natural. Incorporate some of these gestures into your daily communication.

## THE ENERGY FACTOR

Energy is the fuel that drives the car of success. You don't want to run out of gas when you're halfway up the hill. Think back to the last morning that you awoke feeling completely refreshed, like you could conquer the world. Wasn't that a powerful space to be in? That place is exactly where you need to be on the day of the interview—in the zone. This section focuses on ways to unlock your inner energy and present yourself in the best light to the admissions committee.

## Voice and Vocal Variety

Use intonation and inflection in your voice. Speaking in a monotone can be deadly and can put your listeners to sleep. Observe and practice the following rules and exercises to add energy to your voice.

### Rules

1. Make your voice naturally authoritative; speak from the diaphragm.
2. Put your voice on a roller coaster; practice reading from magazines using intonation and inflection.
3. Be aware of your telephone voice; it represents 84% of the emotional impact when people can't see you.
4. Smile when talking on the telephone; people can feel your smile right through the phone.
5. Put your real feelings into your voice.

### Exercises

1. Breathe from the diaphragm. Take in a deep breath from your nose and let it out slowly, stopping to feel the pressure on your diaphragm. This is where a strong voice originates.
2. Project your voice. Try speaking in a normal voice first, and then project your voice so it reaches the back of the room. Try to find the right depth in your voice without straining your vocal chords.
3. Practice varying your pitch and pace. Watch reporters on the network news, as they are masters at using vocal variety. Notice how they emphasize certain words to draw you into the story.

## Words and Nonwords

Energize with words and avoid using nonwords that are meaningless and take away from your message.

### Rules

1. Build your vocabulary, especially with synonyms.
2. Paint word pictures. Create motion and emotion with metaphors.
3. Beware of jargon, especially medical jargon. Say "operating room" instead of "OR."
4. Avoid meaningless nonwords like *ah* and *um*, or words used to stall like *so*, *well*, and *you know*. Replace those words with a silent pause. A properly timed pause adds drama, energy, and power to your message. Try listening to the voice of the famous commentator Paul Harvey on YouTube. He was the master of the pause and made a career out of using the technique. Since many of you will not know who Paul Harvey was Google him, or go to YouTube to find old recordings of his work.

## Listener Involvement

Humans communicate, and books dispense information. Try using the following techniques to add an extra punch to your communication:

### Rules

1. Use a strong opening. Make it visual and energetic by including pauses, action and motion, and joy and laughter.
2. Maintain eye communication. When you enter the room for a group interview, survey your listeners for 3 to 5 seconds, gauge, and adjust.
3. Lean toward your listeners.
4. Create interest by maintaining eye contact and having high energy.

## Use Humor Effectively

President Ronald Reagan was the oldest president in history when he debated Walter Mondale in 1984. The moderator of the debate asked a question about Reagan possibly not having the stamina to be an effective president. Reagan replied, "I am not going to exploit for political purposes my opponent's youth and inexperience." The audience broke out in laughter, and those words changed the entire campaign in Ronald Reagan's favor. You can also Google that debate. Reagan anticipated the "age" question and was prepared with a witty response, which turned out to be the most talked about sentences uttered at the debate.

I do not recommend that you tell jokes at your interview, and remember that fun is better than funny. The goal is not comedy but connection. Find the form of humor that works for you, and be natural. If you feel it's too risky, then avoid the humor.

## Karin's Experience

Let's take a look at what one of my friends and colleagues has to say about her interview experience at Yale University. Karin Augur did not get accepted the first year she applied; however, after making some adjustments, she reapplied the next year and was accepted. Her experience offers a great deal of insight into the interview process and what she learned about herself as a person.

Applying to PA school or any other graduate school can be a very stressful process. Knowing yourself and the profession you are striving to enter are two of the most important factors in the application process. This is particularly evident during the interview. To be absolutely sure that a career as a physician assistant is what you truly desire, you must have an in-depth and intimate knowledge of what a physician assistant does. Conveying that knowledge and your passion for the profession to your interviewer will translate into a successful interview.

When applying to PA school, an impressive application is always important. Once you are granted an interview, demonstrating your attributes in person is even more important. The interviewers are looking for someone with strong character, good communication skills, and focused goals. Even with mediocre qualifications on paper, an impressive interview can significantly increase your chances of being accepted.

My first attempt at PA school proved to be a painful eye-opener. After graduating from one of the top five schools in the country, having earned a BA in biology, I was convinced that earning a Ph.D. for a career in research was my calling in life. After several months working in a cell biology laboratory, I realized this was not my life's dream.

I soon began volunteering at a university emergency department, where I first encountered a physician assistant. Immediately, I knew that career path was one that I would enjoy, and I began preparing to enter PA school immediately. I filled out all of the applications and mentally began to prepare for the interviews. During that year of preparation, I also became engaged to my current husband and found myself preparing for a wedding. As you can imagine, the year was quite hectic and emotionally overwhelming. One by one I heard from each of the schools where I interviewed, and to my utter surprise, I was rejected by all of them. I could not believe it. What had happened? After the initial shock subsided, I soon realized why I was denied acceptance.

Despite being physically present at the various interviews, I was not present in spirit. Besides being distracted by my wedding plans, I had not fully let go of the idea of a career in research. The following year, I not only had to deal with a bruised ego, but I was also forced to take a long, hard look at myself. I continued doing research and volunteering in the emergency department. I decided to start shadowing a PA and realized I had a lot more to learn about the profession. I quickly embraced the idea that, yes, I wanted to be a PA. I focused my energy on improving myself as an applicant. As a result, I was accepted to the school of my choice. I completed the program in two years, finishing second in my class.

Whatever your goals are in life, you must embrace them fully. This is what I learned during my application process. This is exactly what went wrong the first year I applied. Understanding your individual strengths and weaknesses and improving upon them are an excellent way to make yourself a stronger applicant. Learning as much as you can about physician assistants and how you as an individual will satisfy your dreams is as important to your interview as it is to your lifelong happiness.

I think the take-home message in Karin's story is that you really have to do some soul searching and ask yourself what your true motivation is for choosing this career path. Many applicants are just "testing the water" as Karin did her first year applying. It wasn't until she did the work, and realized that research was not for her, that she was able to succeed. Karin is an Ivy league graduate. She had an excellent GPA and test scores. She is also a very intelligent and likeable person. She received many interviews her first year applying, yet she still was not accepted. Her twin sister, also very intelligent and likeable, was my classmate that year, and I know it was a major hit to Karin's ego not to be in our class too. The fact is, although Karin looked great on paper, the interview committee saw that she was not committed enough to become a PA. She did not sell herself as a motivated and passionate applicant that year.

## SUMMARY

In summary, after reading these two interview chapters, you are now well armed to "ace" your PA school interview. Remember to focus on qualities and multipliers when answering your interview questions. The admissions committee already knows the type of applicant they are going to choose, and you want to show them that you have the qualities they're looking for. Remember, it's not about you, it's about them!

Equally important is utilizing high-impact communication skills at your interview. The visual and vocal component of your message that day are just as important as the answers you provide. Be sure to dress appropriately, make eye contact at all times, smile, speak passionately, and use open gestures.

I would strongly recommend signing up for a "mock" interview before your actual interview. This will allow you to practice under fire, and relieve some of that preinterview anxiety. You will also learn what areas of the interview that you need to work on. Many colleges offer "mock" interview services. You want to be sure they understand the PA profession and what type of questions you are going to be asked at the PA school interview. I offer "mock" interview sessions on my website. I've helped hundreds of applicants get accepted, and I'd love to help you too.

# [CHAPTER 9]

# Financial Aid

Now that you have been accepted to PA school, it's time for a reality check relative to paying for your education. For example, if you plan on attending Duke's PA program, you can expect to *invest* approximately $141,027 for your 2-year education. This number includes:

- Tuition
- Books, uniforms, and instruments
- Technology fees
- Food, board, transportation, and miscellaneous
- Health screen
- Background check
- Lab fees
- Student health fees
- Student medical insurance

## THE ALL-IMPORTANT QUESTION: CAN I AFFORD TO GO TO PA SCHOOL?

In my opinion, the real question you should be asking yourself is: Can I afford *not* to go to PA school? If you are really passionate about becoming a PA, then the answer to this question will be an easy one. I left Yale in 1994 with a little over $60,000 worth of debt, which is the equivalent of $97,000 in 2016. My starting salary in 1994 was approximately $45,000, which is equivalent to $77,000 today (consumer price index (CPI),

BLS). However, the starting salary for PAs is currently $98,000, which is $21,000 more than projected by the CPI. The take-home message is that the salaries for the PA professions are growing at a much higher rate than the average professions.

Even though the investment seems quite high—it is just that—an investment. You should think of this investment in terms of what your return on investment will be. For instance, the average earnings potential of a college graduate (bachelor's degree) in 2016 is from $35,000 to $65,000, according to *Money* magazine.

The average salary for a PA (2015) is approximately $98,000, and depending on your specialty area, that number can be as high as $120,000 (BLS). If you do the math, you can see that you will earn almost double the money as a PA than you would in most other professions coming right out of college.

Let's take a look at the math assuming an average starting salary of $98,000 for a PA, and the average starting salary for an "other" profession at $50,000. We will also assume that each profession receives a 3% raise per year. After 10 years, I think you'll be way ahead of the curve if you invest in PA school.

| Year | PA Profession | Other | Difference | |
|------|---------------|-------|------------|---|
| 1 | $98,000 | $50,000 | $48,000 | |
| 2 | 100,940 | 51,500 | 49,440 | |
| 3 | 103,968 | 53,045 | 50,923 | $148,363 |
| 4 | 107,087 | 54,636 | 52,451 | |
| 5 | 110,299 | 56,275 | 54,024 | |
| 6 | 113,607 | 57,963 | 55,644 | |
| 7 | 117,015 | 59,701 | 57,314 | |
| 8 | 120,525 | 61,492 | 59,033 | |
| 9 | 124,140 | 63,336 | 60,804 | |
| 10 | 127,864 | 65,236 | 62,628 | |
| **Total:** | **$1,123,445** | **− 573,184** | **= $550,261** | |

Note that your return on investment for PA school will be realized in less than 3 years. Also note, in 10 years you will earn over one-half million dollars more if you choose the PA route. I would point out that I assumed the raises you would receive as a PA would be the same as for the "other" profession. In reality, a PA with 10-years' experience, who started at $98,000, is very likely to earn much more than $127,000 at that point.

Additionally, Duke's PA program has one of the highest tuition rates/fees. If you attended Campbell's PA program, the tuition would be approximately $50,000 to $60,000 less, and your return on investment would be less than 2 years.

So the real question becomes, can you afford *not* to invest in PA school?

## DECREASING YOUR INVESTMENT

Let's say that you plan on attending Duke's PA program and you realize that the projected investment is going to be $141,000. Is there any way that you can reduce that investment, or get reimbursed for your investment after you graduate? The answer is yes.

If we look at the various expenses listed above, you will notice that there is basically only one way to reduce your expenses while in PA school: food, board, transportation (including parking), books, and miscellaneous. The rest of the items are fixed costs that you cannot do much about.

Let's look at how you may be able to save some money, looking at each one of these items individually.

1. Tuition: You may qualify for reimbursement or a scholarship.
2. Books, uniforms, and instruments: You can buy used books and instruments online. The cost of uniforms will primarily include lab coats.
3. Technology fees: Nonnegotiable.
4. Food, board, transportation, and miscellaneous: I strongly advise to share an apartment with one or two other students, grocery shop at large wholesale chains, minimize eating out, use public transportation to avoid parking fees, or live close enough to walk to school. Be sure to be mindful with all of your expenses and ask yourself: "Do I really need this?"

5. Health screen: You may be able to have this done by your primary care provider, and covered by your insurance.
6. Background check: Nonnegotiable.
7. Lab fees: Nonnegotiable.
8. Student health fees: Nonnegotiable, unless you live in the same town as the program and you are covered by your parents.
9. Student medical insurance: May be negotiable.

# HOW WILL I PAY FOR PA SCHOOL?

Now that we know that the investment for PA school can run in the six-figure range, you may be wondering: "How am I going to pay for this?" In this section I will cover the various financial aid options.

## What Is Financial Aid?

Financial aid is funds provided by federal, state, universities, or external agencies. There are also scholarships and grants (gifts) which require no repayment. Student loans are provided by the federal government at low interest rates. The majority of students pay for their education with student loans.

## The Application Process

The application process for financial aid starts with the completion of the Free Application for Federal Student Aid (FAFSA). The application can be found at FAFSA.gov and completed online. The FAFSA must be completed before you can be considered for federal, state, and university financial aid.

Since you will need tax return data to accomplish the form, I recommend that you use the IRS Data Retrieval tool, which allows you to access the IRS tax return information needed to complete the FAFSA and transfer the data directly into the FAFSA application from the IRS website. This tool is the easiest way to provide your tax data, and it's the best way to ensure that your FAFSA application has accurate tax data.

# What Happens Once the FAFSA Is Completed?

Once you complete the FAFSA application, your financial aid award letter will be determined and sent to the student financial services office (for each program), which may request additional information after receiving it. You will then be notified by email regarding your eligibility for any grants, scholarships, and federal loans. Review all of the information regarding your financial aid award, then either accept or reject the loans.

## Federal Unsubsidized Loans

Securing a federal unsubsidized loan is the way most students will fund their education. Unsubsidized means that the principle payments on the loan do not begin until after graduation, but the interest is *not* paid by the federal government while in school. The student may choose to pay the interest on a monthly basis while in school, or defer the interest payments until after graduation. I recommend the former. If you defer interest payments, the interest will accrue.

To qualify for a federal unsubsidized loan, the FAFSA application must be completed. The interest rate for 2016 to 2017 is 5.31%, fixed. All students automatically qualify for these loans.

The maximum loan amount is $20,500 per year for graduate students. There is a great tool online at studentloans.gov, where you can access a repayment calculator based on the amount of your loans. Although the standard time for repayment is 10 years, there are other options to choose from as far as longer repayment plans.

## Payment Plans and Loan Options

You PA program may offer a monthly payment plan to pay part, or all, of your educational expenses. There are obvious benefits to begin making payments early, but this option is probably not going to be very realistic for most of you.

Some other loan options include private alternative loans from various venders like Sallie Mae, Wells Fargo, Citizens bank, to name a few. These loans require a credit review and have variable or fixed interest rates. You can apply for these loans online and you can do a side-by-side comparison at elmselect.com.

Federal graduate PLUS loans are another option. The interest rate for PLUS loans in 2016 is 6.31% (fixed). A PLUS loan is separate from the $20,5000 per year from the federal subsidized loans, but they are a good option for PA students. The student can apply for these loans online at studentloans.gov and receive approval in a matter of a few minutes. The loan amount is determined by the Department of Education, and your credit score will be a factor in the decision. You may use an endorser on these loans.

## Tuition Reimbursement, Private Scholarships, and Other Sources

Some other sources of tuition assistance include private outside scholarships, local and national, which you can find on the program's website for a listing of available scholarships.

There are also federal grant programs like National Health Service Corps (NHSC), Indian Health Service (IHS), Department of Health and Human Services scholarships for health profession students from disadvantaged backgrounds, state programs, and through the American Academy of Physician Assistant (AAPA).

The National Health Service Corps is an excellent program that covers tuition and provides you with a monthly stipend. You will incur a 2-year obligation to a designated (underserved) location. You will be given several sites to select from throughout the country. You will be required to contact those sites for availability and negotiate a salary. Four hundred NHSC awards are provided each year. To qualify, you must accomplish a questionnaire and an application.

Contact information:

Contact: NHSC Scholarships
Division of Applications and Awards
5600 Fishers Lane, Room 8A-55
Rockville, Maryland, 20857
(315) 594-4400
Website: hrsa.gov

The Indian Health Service is another alternative. The IHS requires a minimum 2-year obligation in return for 2 years of financial support. Priority is given to Native American students, but others may apply.

> Contact: IHS Scholarship Office
> (800) 962-2817
> Website: ihs.gov

The Department of Health and Human Services also offers scholarships for health professional students from disadvantaged backgrounds. Applicants must be able to prove financial need and prove enrollment or acceptance to a PA program. Applicants must also be full-time students.

> Contact: federalgrantswire.com/scholarships-for-health-professionals

There are some state programs available that include loan forgiveness. You will be required to work at a designated site in an underserved area and receive up to $20,000 in loan forgiveness.

You should also look into the Health Profession Shortage Area (HPSA) program, which provides loans at a dollar-for-dollar match for educational loans.

Many state/constituent chapters of the AAPA offer scholarship programs for PA students. Contact your state chapter for availability.

## VA Military Benefits

The Yellow Ribbon GI Education Enhancement Program (Yellow Ribbon Program) is a provision of the Post-9/11 GI Bill that allows veterans to attend private schools and graduate programs costing more than the state tuition cap. Under the program, participating PA programs must offer a veterans-only scholarship which the VA will then match up to the full cost of tuition and fees.

For example, in the District of Columbia the Post 9/11 GI Bill will only provide $3,000 toward tuition/fees. George Washington University, however, the college to accept the WWII GI Bill, has signed up for the Yellow Ribbon Program and agreed to contribute $18,000 toward a veteran's tuition/fees. The VA will match that $18,000 contribution under the Yellow Ribbon Program. A veteran attending George Washington University will receive a full ride, up to $39,000/year toward their tuition and fees.

## Useful Resources

U.S. Department of Veterans Affairs: Post 9/11 GI Bill
(gibill.va.gov/benefits/post_911_gibill/index.html)

U.S. Department of Veterans Affairs: Yellow Ribbon Program
(benefits.va.gov/GIBILL/yellow_ribbon/Yellow_Ribbon_Info_Schools.asp)

NAICU: Outreach to Veterans
(Naicu.edu/special_initiatives/gibill/outreach_to_veterans/)

NAICU: About the GI Bill
(naicu.edu/special_initiatives/gibill/about/)

**The individual PA program's financial aid office.**

# [CHAPTER 10]

# The Internet for PA School Applicants

The Internet provides a wealth of knowledge for those interested in the PA profession. Whether you want to research a particular PA program, gain more knowledge of the PA profession itself, learn about national and state issues relative to the PA profession, or join a PA forum to interact with other applicants and PA school faculty members, it's all available on the Internet.

Every PA program in the United States has a website that provides all of the information that you will need to know about that particular program. You can find things like admissions requirements, the curriculum, PANCE rates, financial aid, student societies, mission and vision statements, number of students applying, number of students accepted, and the average statistics of accepted students.

The Internet also provides a variety of organizational and personal websites for PA school applicants. My personal website, andrewrodican. com, is exclusively designed for PA school applicants who want to maximize their chances of getting into PA school. Here are some of the highlights from my website:

- Selecting a PA program
- The CASPA application
- The essay
- The interview
- My coaching programs
- *U.S. News & World Report* best PA program rankings

- The #1 reason PA school applicants get rejected
- My interview with an ABC affiliate station
- PA school interview video
- Link to AAPA website
- Link to state/constituent chapters of the AAPA
- Link to CASPA FAQs
- List of programs utilizing rolling admissions
- Nurse practitioner versus PA
- PANCE rates for each PA program
- All of my books for sale

# WEBSITES

## American Academy of Physician Assistants (AAPA) (aapa.org)

The American Academy of Physician Assistants (AAPA) is the only national organization that represents physician assistants in all specialties and employment settings. Membership includes physician assistants, physician assistant students, physician assistant hopefuls, and those interested in supporting the physician assistant profession. The AAPA's website provides volumes of information for PA school applicants, and it's a "must view" website. The following information and resources are available on the website:

- Information about the AAPA
- How to join the AAPA
- PA organizations
- About PAs
- Member benefits and services
- Continuing Medical Education (CME) and clinical issues
- Reimbursement issues
- Professional practice issues
- Employment and employer's guide
- "Hot topics" relevant to the PA profession
- PA salary reports

- National issues facing the PA profession
- Current events
- AAPA national survey results
- Events
- News & publications
- Press releases

## Physician Assistant Education Association (PAEA) (paeaonline.org)

The Physician Assistant Education Association (PAEA) is the only national organization representing physician assistant educational programs in the United States. Currently, all of the accredited programs in the country are members of the association. PAEA provides services for faculty at its member programs, as well as to applicants, students, and other stakeholders.

The PAEA also provides a searchable PA programs directory, and the CASPA application.

## CASPA Application FAQ Page (caspaonline.org)

Everything you need to know about accomplishing the CASPA application is located on this page; I mean everything! Be sure to frequent this page if you have any questions relevant to the CASPA application.

## Association of Postgraduate Physician Assistant Programs (appap.org)

The Association of Postgraduate Physician Assistant Programs (APPAP) provides educational, professional, and informational support to PAs. This is a website where you can find a listing of all of the postgraduate PA programs in the country. See Appendix 1 for a listing of current postgraduate programs.

## Journal of the American Academy of Physician Assistants (JAAPA) (jaapa.com)

This is the official journal of the AAPA and is clinically oriented, geared toward practicing PAs and PA students. In addition to clinical articles, the journal frequently reports on issues relevant to the PA profession. The journal also provides a listing of job opportunities, which can be motivational for aspiring PAs.

## Central Application Service for Physician Assistants (CASPA) (caspaonline.org)

The Central Application Service for Physician Assistants (CASPA) offers a web-based application service (used by the majority of PA programs) that allows PA school applicants to apply to multiple, participating, PA programs, by completing a single online application.

## Federal Student Aid (fafsa.ed.gov)

The Federal Student Aid website provides information relevant to financial aid available from the U.S. Department of Education. The Federal Student Aid programs are the largest source of student aid in the United States, providing more than $60 billion a year in grants, loans, and work-study assistance. Here you'll find help for every stage of the financial aid process, whether you're in school or out of school.

## U.S. Department of Veterans Affairs—Yellow Ribbon Program (benefits.va.gov/gibill/yellow_ribbon.asp)

The Yellow Ribbon GI Education Enhancement Program (Yellow Ribbon Program) is a provision of the Post-9/11 GI Bill that allows veterans to attend private schools and graduate programs costing more than the state tuition cap. Under the program, participating colleges and universities must offer a veterans-only scholarship which the VA will then match up to the full cost of tuition and fees.

## Accreditation Review Commission on Education for the Physician Assistant (ARC-PA) (arc-pa.org)

The Accreditation Review Commission on Education for the Physician Assistant (ARC-PA) is the accrediting agency that protects the interests of the public and the PA profession by defining the standards for PA education and evaluating PA educational programs in the territorial United States to ensure their compliance with those standards.

## National Commission of Certification of Physician Assistants (NCCPA) (nccpa.net)

The National Commission of Certification of Physician Assistants (NCCPA) is the only credentialing organization for physician assistants in the United States. Established as a not-for-profit organization in 1975, the NCCPA is dedicated to ensuring that certified physician assistants meet established standards of knowledge and clinical skills on entry into practice and throughout their careers. Every U.S. state, the District of Columbia, and the U.S. territories rely on the NCCPA certification as a criterion for licensure or regulation of physician assistants. The NCCPA has currently certified over 100,000 PAs.

## PA Forum (physicianassistantforum.com)

The PA Forum is a resource center established for PAs, PA students, and Pre-PAs in 1988. There are multiple discussion groups on the PA Forum:
   News & Announcements

- Announcements

Professional Physician Assistant

- Professional PA General Discussion
- Medical Billing and Coding
- Specialties
- Military
- State Specific Discussion
- Physician Assistant Residency
- Physician Assistant Owned Practice
- Contracts, Negotiations, and Malpractice

International Physician Assistant Forum

- International Physician Assistant
- International Physician Assistant Schools

Physician Assistant Student Forums

- PA Student General Discussion
- Shadowing Opportunities
- Clinical Rotations
- PANCE/PANRE
- Financial Aid
- Textbooks & Medical Equipment for Sale

Pre-PA

- Pre-PA General Discussion
- Physician Assistant Schools
- CASPA
- Personal Statements

Miscellaneous

- The Recovery Room
- Website Support

PA Blogs

A listing of the best PA blogs of 2016

- doximity.com
- https://blog.doximity.com/articles/best-pa-blogs-of-2016

I strongly recommend that all Pre-PAs visit the PA Forum and sign up for membership. The PA Forum is truly a valuable resource, and it's free!

# [CHAPTER 11]

# Frequently Asked Questions

After being involved with coaching PA school applicants since 1996, I have come to know about some of the most commonly asked questions by PA school applicants. In this chapter I am going to share these questions and provide the answers.

## QUESTION #1: DO I HAVE A CHANCE?

Applicants routinely post this question on the PA Forum, along with their statistics (GPA, GRE, clinical experience) expecting people to respond with a yes? or a no? The problem is, without reading the applicant's essay, or evaluating their interview skills, it is impossible to answer this question! A more appropriate question would be, "Am I a competitive applicant?"

The essay is your ticket to the interview, and a well-written essay can transcend less than average grades or medical experience. Even then, if you do make it to the interview, and you don't make that critical emotional connection with the committee, you will have no chance of being accepted.

So I advise applicants to stay focused, and do the work necessary to become the perfect applicant before you apply. Then I recommend writing a "killer" essay, and learn how to "ace" the PA school interview.

# QUESTION #2: WHAT CAN I DO TO IMPROVE MY APPLICATION?

That's an easy question to answer.

First, forget about the published "minimum" requirements on a program's website. The perfect applicant will exceed the minimum requirements with respect to GPA, GRE scores, and health care experience.

Second, review Chapter 2 for real numbers from first-year "accepted" PA students. These are the numbers you should strive for, because this is what the competition will be bringing to the table.

Third, if you review the numbers in Chapter 2, and you fall short in any area, work hard to improve your numbers before you apply.

Finally, if you aren't a competitive applicant yet, consider waiting another year to strengthen your application before you apply. In the grand scheme of things, waiting one more year will not make a difference 10 years down the road. Strengthening your application may also be the difference between getting into the PA school of your choice, or settling for a school that you're not too excited about, or where you may not be a good fit.

# QUESTION #3: DO YOU HAVE ANY ADVICE FOR REAPPLICANTS?

Yes! The first thing the admissions committee is going to do when they review your application, and realize you are a reapplicant, is to see what you've done to improve your application from last year.

Attempt find out why you were not accepted last year. This may be hard to do sometimes, as you're likely to receive the standard response: "We had a lot of competitive applicants this year, and unfortunately we only have a limited number of slots available. We cannot accept everyone." This information is meaningless. The answer is not personal to you, and it doesn't help you prepare to improve your application for the next cycle.

If you made it to the interview, and did not get accepted, chances are you did not interview well, and you will need to work on your interview skills.

In any case, there a several things that you must do to demonstrate to the committee (this year) that you are a serious, passionate, and motivated applicant:

- Continue to take upper level sciences course, and get A's
- Continue to gain hands-on medical experience

- Continue to shadow PAs
- Continue to stay current with the PA profession by frequenting the AAPA website and your state chapter of the AAPA website
- Try contacting students from the program and get a sense for the qualities the program is looking for in accepted applicants. What does the program value most?
- Review the mission statement of the program, and be sure to make yourself a good fit for that program. For example, if the program values community service, get some volunteer experience.

More than likely you are going to be asked, directly, at your interview: "What have you done to improve your application this year?" If you do the work mentioned above, you are going to come across as a motivated and passionate applicant. If you don't, you'll be looked at as someone who may be just testing the waters, and as someone who really is not invested in becoming a PA.

## QUESTION #4: HOW DO I GET MEDICAL EXPERIENCE? I'M A FULL-TIME STUDENT AND I DON'T HAVE MUCH FREE TIME

Without sounding too direct...no, let me be direct: figure it out! If you can't work part-time and go to school full-time, how are you going to handle a rigorous PA program? Are you not able to multi-task? Are you not able to handle stress? Are you not motivated enough to get the necessary experience to become a competitive applicant? These are just some of the questions an admissions committee will consider if you apply to PA school with little, or no medical experience.

Unlike young medical school applicants who are not expected/required to have direct patient contact hours, there's a totally different philosophy with respect to PA school applicants. The PA profession is not an entry-level profession. Remember, the first PAs were former Navy corpsman who had 3 or 4 years of combat medical experience. Competitive applicants will have 2,500 to 3,000 hours of hands-on direct patient contact. Why would you think that you would be a competitive applicant without medical experience?

PA school is really not for the very young applicant, as it is very difficult to acquire patient contact hours when you are in college, or especially if you decide on this career path later on in college. The mean age of a first-year PA school student is 26. There are those applicants who do get accepted to PA school right out of college, but I would say these applicants are more the exception than the rule.

I don't mean to discourage the younger applicants reading this book; I just want to be realistic about the application process, and what it takes to be a competitive applicant. Those applicants who are young, but mature, seem to figure out a way to get the experience and get accepted.

## QUESTION #5: HOW DO I FIND A PA TO SHADOW?

Great question! Shadowing PAs is a requirement for applying to PA school. How would you know that you want to become a PA if you haven't shadowed a PA? However, with the advent of HIPPA regulations, it has become much more difficult for PA school applicants to find PAs to shadow. It is almost impossible at many hospitals.

Fear not! The best way to find PAs to shadow is by joining your state chapter of the AAPA, attending local meetings, and networking with the PAs you encounter at those meetings. Most PAs are very willing to give back to the profession by allowing applicants to shadow them. We all had to find PAs to shadow and we appreciate the need for you to have to do the same thing. If you can find a group of PAs that you can meet face-to-face, and network with them, you will have a much better chance of being successful than if you simply contact random PAs in your area.

Many state chapters of the AAPA also have lists of PAs in the state who are willing to allow applicants to shadow them. Give the organization a call and see if they can help.

## QUESTION #6: I HAVE A LOWER THAN AVERAGE GPA, WHAT CAN I DO TO BECOME MORE COMPETITIVE AS AN APPLICANT?

Chances are that if you have a low GPA after finishing undergrad, you would need to take a lot more classes to move your GPA into a competitive range (depending on how low it is).

When I served on the admissions committee, I looked more at the applicant's *trend* versus the absolute GPA number. So, if you have a lower than average GPA, begin taking some upper level graduate science courses: genetics, chemistry, and physiology. Be sure to get A's in those classes to demonstrate to the committee that you can handle the difficult didactic phase of the PA program. If you take five or six science courses and do well, you may be able to compensate for your overall lower GPA.

## QUESTION #7: WHO SHOULD I (IDEALLY) ASK TO PROVIDE MY LETTERS OF RECOMMENDATION (LOR)?

I always recommend that you, first, look at the program's requirements to see if they specify who they want LORs from. Typically, I would recommend that you obtain an LOR from at least one PA. The other two LORs should come from an individual who knows you well enough to comment, specifically, on the qualities you have that would be valuable as a PA school student and as a graduate PA. Usually a professor, supervisor, or an MD is appropriate.

Be sure to consider the person you are asking carefully. If it's getting late in the CASPA application process, and you are missing one LOR in order to verify your CASPA application, would you feel comfortable calling that person on the phone and asking them to get the LOR submitted ASAP. If the answer is no, don't select that person to write your LOR. It may be tempting to ask a "big shot" to write your LOR because you think her name will carry a lot of weight with the program. However, her name will be meaningless if she fails to submit your LOR on time, and you don't feel comfortable calling her to get her moving!

## QUESTION #8: HOW MANY PROGRAMS SHOULD I APPLY TO?

With the advent of the CASPA application, it is now easier than ever to apply to multiple programs by accomplishing a single, online application. The more programs you apply to, the better your odds are of getting invited to interview. Does that mean you should apply to 40 programs? Absolutely not! From my observations, I find that the majority of PA school applicants apply to anywhere from 5 to 15 programs. You should select the programs that you choose to apply to be centered on the fact that you are a good fit for that program, and not out of convenience or because you want to use the "shotgun" approach.

# QUESTION #9: IF I'M ASKED; "HAVE YOU APPLIED TO OTHER PROGRAMS?" BY THE ADMISSIONS COMMITTEE, HOW SHOULD I ANSWER?

This is a legitimate question, and a concern of many applicants whom I work with on mock interviews. Many applicants fear that if they tell the admissions committee they've applied to several programs, that information will somehow diminish their chances of being accepted to that program. The fact is, if you are a serious applicant, motivated and passionate about becoming a PA, you are *expected* to apply to several programs.

If you admit to applying to only one program, the committee will question your motivation for wanting to become a PA. Why would you put all of your eggs in one basket if you're really motivated to become a PA?

If you apply to only one program, like Duke, your odds of acceptance may be less than 1%! With those odds, you really don't appear to be someone who really cares if they get accepted or not. Perhaps you're just testing the water?

On the other hand, if you apply to 40 programs, you are going to appear unfocused and desperate. What could be the common denominator between 40 programs? How will you explain why you've chosen the programs you have? What do they all have in common? Good luck with that one.

The bottom line is that you will not diminish your chances of acceptance if you tell the truth! ADCOM members have been doing this for a very long time and they know, and expect, applicants to apply to multiple programs.

# QUESTION #10: WHAT IF THEY ASK AT MY INTERVIEW: "WHICH PROGRAM IS YOUR TOP CHOICE?"

This question can be extremely anxiety-provoking. What if the program you're interviewing with is *not* your top choice program? Do you lie, and tell the ADCOM it is? It's never a good idea to lie at an interview, but you can put a positive *spin* on your answer.

Think about this...chances are that if you are being interviewed at XYZ PA program, you probably haven't been accepted to your top choice yet; unless XYZ is your top choice and the answer to this question is easy.

Technically, even if XYZ PA program is not your top choice, it is your only choice at the time of your interview, unless you've been accepted elsewhere. If you've been accepted elsewhere and you are satisfied with attending that program, you wouldn't need to interview at XYZ. So you can honestly answer that XYZ is your top choice. Why? Because it is your only choice, right now!

## QUESTION #11: HOW IMPORTANT IS THE SCIENCE GPA WHEN LOOKING AT POTENTIAL STUDENTS, AND, IF NOT PROVIDED ONLINE, WHAT IS THE MINIMUM OR RECOMMENDED SCIENCE GPA FOR STUDENTS TO HAVE?

Typically, the medical core or prerequisite GPA can sometimes paint a more accurate picture of the applicant's performance in the sciences. Many program's use an applicant's performance in prerequisite courses, especially in the upper level biologies and chemistries, to "predict" if the student would be able to handle the demanding and rigorous PA curriculum. Many programs recommend an applicant have at least a 3.2 or higher prerequisite GPA to be competitive with the applicant pool. You will find the average prerequisite GPA for most programs to be between 3.4 and 3.6.

## QUESTION #12: WHAT KIND OF MEDICAL EXPERIENCE IS PREFERRED, INCLUDING THOSE FROM THE LIST OF SUGGESTIONS ONLINE?

On average, most incoming students will have a certification as a certified nursing assistant (CAN), EMT/Paramedic, medical assistant (MA), physical therapy assistant, or phlebotomist. Programs prefer applicants have paid experience, but many students accumulate all of their hours through shadowing a PA and a physician. Realize that not all PA programs accept shadowing as a way to fulfill the clinical experience hours, but you will find that many programs strongly recommend shadowing in addition to paid hours.

Shadowing is a great way for applicants to get a feel for the role of the PA in clinical practice, and also to help the applicant understand what they are getting themselves into. I think most programs would say that the purpose of having clinical experience is exactly for the reasons listed above. Many programs list acceptable experience requirements on their websites.

## QUESTION #13: IS RESEARCH RECOMMENDED FOR APPLICANTS, OR IS CLINICAL EXPERIENCE ENOUGH?

Research is not something most programs put a lot of emphasis on simply because the role of the PA is not really research driven. That being said, there are many PAs who contribute to medical research, but the goal of most programs is to produce the best mid-level providers through clinically relevant teaching. This is where quality clinical experience prior to PA school is so beneficial. Of course a research background may be useful when completing the graduate research paper that is part of the curriculum, but this can be successfully completed without a strong research background. You may find that many medical programs put more emphasis on research more so than PA programs.

## QUESTION #14: DO MOST STUDENTS TAKE OUT LOANS FOR TUITION? IS THERE ANY FINANCIAL AID AVAILABLE, FROM THE COLLEGE OR FROM OUTSIDE OF THE COLLEGE?

I would estimate about 95% of students will finance their tuition, expenses for the program (equipment and books), and living expenses through student loans. No PA program will ever encourage students to have an outside job while attending PA school. In fact, most programs do not allow students to work outside of school.

See the financial aid section in this book (Chapter 9) for various options on loans, grants, and scholarships.

# QUESTION #15: IS IT COMMON FOR POTENTIAL APPLICANTS TO TAKE TIME OFF AFTER UNDERGRADUATE SCHOOL TO ACCUMULATE CLINICAL EXPERIENCE?

This is a very common question. There are a wide variety of students who are right out of their undergraduate program, some who have taken 1 to 5 years off, and some who are now in the midst of changing their career. Preference is *not* given to applicants who have taken time off between undergraduate and PA school, but sometimes you can find that "real life" experience may be beneficial in adjusting to PA school and being more prepared for the profession you're about to enter. I always stress that applicants should not attend/apply to PA school until they feel they are ready. If your preparation requires time off in between graduation and PA school, especially to accumulate clinical experience hours, I would strongly recommend taking time off. This is especially true for younger applicants who may be fresh out of college and have no clinical experience at all.

# QUESTION #16: WHAT ARE SOME OF THE MOST COMMON MISTAKES INDIVIDUALS MAKE WHEN APPLYING TO PA SCHOOL?

Here are five major mistakes:

1. *Writing an ineffective personal statement.* You must be able to communicate in your personal statement that you understand what you are getting yourself into—meaning you understand the role of the physician assistant, how PAs benefit the health care system, and what experiences (clinically) have led you to believe that the PA profession is a good fit for you. One common opening sentence for many applicants is something along the lines of "Ever since I was five-years-old I played with my dad's doctor's kit or read my mom's anatomy book..." ADCOMs see this so often, the words are meaningless and unrealistic. Be unique. Make sure to have someone else read your personal statement before you upload it into your CASPA application. Having a typo or grammatical error in your essay could be the "kiss of death" for your candidacy.

2. *Selecting the wrong people to write your letters of recommendation.* Find three people who will provide you with GOOD letters of recommendation. I realize that it is impossible to predict what another person will write on your behalf, but make sure they can elaborate on your skills and potential as a PA. Believe it or not, there are some physicians who've submitted an LOR with only one sentence! See Appendix 5 for more detailed information.

3. *Not meeting all of the prerequisite requirements before applying.* Make sure that you meet all of the requirements for the program(s) to which you are applying.

4. *Not meeting the selection criteria.* Most programs have a minimum recommended overall GPA of 3.0 or higher, prerequisite GPA between 3.2 and 3.4, clinical experience requirements, and at least a GRE score of 297 to 300. Some applicants hope programs make exceptions for their past performance. With the number of PA school applicants applying each year, programs take the most competitive applicants based on meeting the selection factors above. Why would a program settle for less?

5. *Applying too late.* Many applicants wait until October through December to start the CASPA application. Each year CASPA opens in mid-April for entry into the next year's class so it is important to start as early as you can. Additionally, as mentioned in the CASPA chapter, many programs have rolling admissions, so it's first come, first served at those programs. The class will probably be filled by October. See Appendix 4 for a current listing of programs that utilize rolling admissions. Keep in mind this list is current as of 2016, and is certainly subject to change.

# QUESTION #17: I AM A FOREIGN MEDICAL GRADUATE (FMG), WILL MY CLINICAL EXPERIENCE COUNT TOWARD A PROGRAM'S CLINICAL REQUIREMENTS?

Some programs count foreign MD hours toward their clinical experience requirement. Be sure to check with your program(s) before applying. Realize, however, that FMGs will still have to meet all of the academic prerequisites to be considered.

## QUESTION #18: IS THERE A PREFERRED MAJOR THAT WILL MAKE ME A MORE COMPETITIVE APPLICANT?

If you are in undergraduate school, I would recommend choosing a biology or chemistry major if you definitely know you will be applying to PA school. The reason for this is that you are likely to meet all of the prerequisite requirements for most programs by the time you graduate. You will find that if your major is in business or psychology, for example, then you will need to take additional courses after completing your degree to meet the PA program prerequisite classes (i.e., General Chemistry I & II, Organic Chemistry I & II, Anatomy and Physiology, Biochemistry)

Having said that, if you are a career changer, and your major is not in a science, it doesn't mean you cannot apply to PA school. You will just need to take the prerequisites and if you do well, you will be as competitive as any other applicant.

## QUESTION #19: MY MOTHER IS A PA, WOULD THIS HURT ME OR HELP ME IN REGARDS TO APPLYING TO PA SCHOOL?

Great question! I can't see how your mom being a PA would hurt your chances. If anything, her being a PA should be a good resource for you to understand the profession better and maybe she has recommendations on places to get your clinical hours. She's also "been there, done that" with PA school. She could provide great support as you go through PA school!

On the other hand, you will need to have your application and goal to become a PA stand on its own. Don't project a sense of entitlement, and be sure to express why *you* want to be a PA. You might come off as a bit immature if you cannot provide a clear reason why you are choosing this path, and your answer better not be, "Because my mom is a PA."

## QUESTION #20: I'M AN OLDER APPLICANT, WILL THAT HURT MY CHANCES OF ACCEPTANCE?

Never think that you are too old for PA school. Nontraditional students can bring a lot to the table. If you're going back to retake classes, be sure to do well in the prerequisite coursework. More than any other factor, the admissions committee wants to be assured that *any* applicant will be able to handle the rigorous science coursework in PA school.

Additionally, programs are looking for specific qualities in applicants applying to PA school. Those qualities are not necessarily relevant to the medical field, and many older applicants have the transferable skills needed to fulfill those qualities.

If you have any questions that you would like me to personally answer, feel free to email me at andyrodican@gmail.com. I would be more than happy to help!

# APPENDIX 1

# List of Postgraduate PA Programs

1. Albany Medical Center PA Post-Graduate Fellowship in Emergency Medicine
2. Albert Einstein Medical Center Physician Assistant Emergency Medicine Residency
3. Arrowhead Orthopaedic's—PA Orthopaedic Surgery Residency Program
4. Arrowhead Regional Medical Center—CEP America Paid Emergency Medicine PA Fellowship—Southern California
5. Bassett Healthcare Multispecialty Surgical—Postgraduate Physician Assistant Program
6. Baylor College of Medicine Emergency Medicine Physician Assistant Fellowship
7. Carilion Clinic Advanced Practitioner Fellowship in Orthopedic Surgery
8. Carilion Clinic Department of Emergency Medicine—Carilion Clinic Advanced Practice Clinician
9. Carolinas Healthcare System Acute Care/Critical Care Fellowship Program
10. Carolinas Healthcare System Primary Care and Urgent Care Fellowship: Pediatrics, Internal Medicine, Family Medicine, Urgent Care and Pediatric Urgent Care
11. Carolinas Healthcare System Specialty Care Fellowship: Cardiology, Urology, and Behavioral Health
12. Children's Hospital of Philadelphia—Neonatal Physician Assistant Program

13. Dartmouth—Hitchcock Medical Center Cardiothoracic Surgery Physician Assistant Post Graduate Residency Program

14. DMC Orthopedic Surgery and Sports Medicine PA Fellowship

15. Duke University Medical Center—PA Surgical Residency Duke University Medical Center

16. Emory Critical Care Center NP/PA Post Graduate Residency Program

17. EVMS Physician Assistant Fellowship in Emergency Medicine— Emergency Medicine

18. Hartford Healthcare PA Surgery—Critical Care Residency Program—Residency and Surgery

19. Hospital Medicine PA Fellowship at Regions Hospital

20. Illinois Bone and Joint Institute—Postgraduate PA Orthopedic Residency Program

21. Intermountain Medical Center Trauma and Surgical Critical Care—Postgraduate Fellowship for PAs and NPs

22. Iowa Emergency Medicine Physician Assistant Residency Program

23. Jane R. Perlman NP/PA Fellowship in Emergency Medicine

24. Johns Hopkins Bayview Medical Center—Emergency Medicine PA Residency

25. Johns Hopkins Hospital—Postgraduate Critical Care Residency for PAs

26. Johns Hopkins Hospital—Postgraduate Surgical Residency for PAs

27. Marquette University—Aurora Health Postgraduate Physician Assistant Emergency Medicine Program—Emergency Medicine Program

28. Mayo Clinic—Mayo Clinic Arizona PA Fellowship in Otolaryngology

29. Mayo Clinic Arizona Postgraduate Fellowship in Hospital Internal Medicine—with optional hematology/Oncology and Critical Care Medicine Tracks

30. Mercer-piedmont Heart Physician Assistant Residency in Advanced Cardiology

31. Methodist Debakey Heart and Vascular Surgery PA Residency Program—Methodist Debakey Heart and Vascular Surgery PA Residency

32. Montefiore Medical Center—Albert Einstein College of Medicine—Postgraduate Residency in Surgery for PAs

33. Montefiore Medical Center—Postgraduate Ob-Gyn Residency

34. Nationwide Children's Hospital Child and Adolescent Psychiatry Physician Assistant Postgraduate Training Program

35. New York Presbyterian Hospital—Weill Cornell Medical Center—PA Residency in Internal Medicine

36. Norwalk Hospital—Norwalk/Yale PA Surgical Residency Program

37. Regions Hospital—Emergency Medicine PA Residency Program

38. SJMH Residency in Cardiothoracic Critical Care

39. St. Joseph Mercy Hospital—PA Residency in Cardiothoracic Surgery

40. St. Luke's University Health Network—Critical Care and Emergency Medicine Advanced Practitioner (PA/NP) Fellowship

41. Staten Island University Hospital Physician Assistant Post Graduate Fellowship in Emergency Medicine

42. Team Health EMAPC Fellowship—Emergency Medicine

43. Texas Children's Hospital Surgery Physician Assistant Fellowship

44. The University of Texas MD Anderson Cancer Center—Postgraduate PA Fellowship Program in Oncology

45. UCSF Fresno Emergency Medicine PA Residency

46. UCSF Fresno Orthopedic Surgery PA Residency Program

47. University of Florida PA Surgical Residency Program

48. University of Iowa Carver College of Medicine—PA Residency Psychiatry

49. University of Kentucky—University of Kentucky PA Residency in Neonatology

50. University of Missouri—Post Graduate Acute Care Residency

51. University of Missouri Postgraduate Emergency Medicine PA Residency

52. UPMC Advanced Practice Provider Postgraduate Surgical Residency Program—Surgery

53. UT Southwest Medical Center at Dallas—Physician Assistant Urology Residency Program

54. WakeMed Health and Hospitals—PA Residency in Trauma Critical Care, and Surgery

55. Winthrop University Hospital—PA Postgraduate Surgical Critical Care Program
56. Yale New-Haven Hospital Emergency Medicine PA Residency Program

    Postgraduate PA Programs Website: (aapa.org/post-graduate-pa-programs/programs/)

# The Tournament Draw Technique Format

Make a list of all the eight most important items you will need to accomplish before applying to PA school:

1. _____

2. _____

3. _____

4. _____

5. _____

6. _____

7. _____

8. _____

Now place those items in the first round of the chart below. Use the Tournament Draw Technique to come up with the winner: the first item you need to accomplish.

| Round 1 | Round 2 | Round 3 | Winner |
|---------|---------|---------|--------|
| 1. | | | |
| 2. | | | |
| 3. | | | |
| 4. | | | Winner |
| 5. | | | |
| 6. | | | |
| 7. | | | |
| 8. | | | |

# PA Programs' First-Time PANCE Rates as of 2016

| PA Program | First-Time Pass/Fail Rates |
|---|---|
| Adventist University of Health Sciences | TBD |
| Albany Medical College | 97% |
| Alderson-Broaddus University | 69% (2013) |
| Anne Arundel Community College | 98% |
| Arcadia University | 100% |
| Arizona School of Health Sciences | Not Listed |
| Augsburg College | 99% |
| Baldwin Wallace University | 100% (1 yr.) |
| Barry University | 91% |
| Bay Path University | 82%–87% (2014–2015) |
| Baylor College of Medicine | 97% |
| Bethel University | 100% (2015) |

*(Continued)*

| PA Program | First-Time Pass/Fail Rates |
|---|---|
| Bethel University, Tennessee | 96% |
| Boston University | TBD |
| Bryant University | TBD |
| Butler University | 96% |
| Campbell University | 94% (2013–2015) |
| Carroll University | 97% |
| Case Western Reserve University | TBD |
| CCNY Sophie Davis School of Biomedical Education | 95% |
| Central Michigan University | 96% |
| Chapman University | TBD |
| Charles R. Drew University | TBD |
| Chatham University | 94% |
| Christian Brothers University | 70% (2 yr.) |
| Clarkson University | 100% (2 yr.) |
| College of Saint Joseph | TBD |
| College of Saint Scholastica | TBD |
| Concordia University | 86% (2015) |
| Cornell University | 90% (2003–2007) |
| CUNY York College | 80% |
| Cuyahoga Community College/Cleveland State University | 88% |
| D'Youville College | 88% |
| Daemen College | 98% (2009–2013) |
| Des Moines University | 97% |

*(Continued)*

| PA Program | First-Time Pass/Fail Rates |
| --- | --- |
| DeSales University | 100% |
| Dominican University | TBD |
| Dominican University of California | TBD |
| Drexel University | 95% (2009–2013) |
| Duke University Medical Center | 96% |
| Duquesne University | 92% |
| East Carolina University | 99% |
| Eastern Michigan University | 100% (2015) |
| Eastern Virginia Medical School | 97% |
| Elon University | 97% (2015–2016) |
| Emory University | 95% |
| FIU Herbert Wertheim College of Medicine | TBD |
| Francis Marion University | TBD |
| Franklin College | TBD |
| Franklin Pierce University | 91% (2012–2015) |
| Gannon University | 91% (2010–2014) |
| Gardner Webb University | TBD |
| George Washington University | 94% |
| Georgia Regents University | 95% |
| Grand Valley State University | 100% |
| Hardin-Simmons University | TBD |
| Harding University | 90% (2009–2014) |
| Heritage University | TBD |
| High Point University | TBD |

*(Continued)*

| PA Program | First-Time Pass/Fail Rates |
|---|---|
| Hofstra University | 98% |
| Howard University | 86% |
| Idaho State University | 96% |
| Indiana State University | 90% (2013–2015) |
| Indiana University School of Health and Rehab Sciences | 90% (2015) |
| Interservice | 97% |
| James Madison University | 94% |
| Jefferson College of Health Sciences | 98% |
| Johnson & Wales University | 100% (2016) |
| Kean University | TBD |
| Keiser University | 85% |
| Kettering College | 99% (2013–2015) |
| King's College | 94% |
| Lake Erie College | TBD |
| Le Moyne College | 94% |
| Lenoir-Rhyne University | TBD |
| Lincoln Memorial | 91% |
| Lock Haven University | 96% |
| Loma Linda University | 94% |
| Long Island University | 90% |
| Louisiana State University, New Orleans | 100% (2015) |
| Louisiana State University, Shreveport | Not Reported |
| Lynchburg College | TBD |

*(Continued)*

| PA Program | First-Time Pass/Fail Rates |
| --- | --- |
| Marietta College | 94% |
| Marist College | TBD |
| Marquette University | 100% |
| Marshall B. Ketchum University | TBD |
| Mary Baldwin College | TBD |
| Marywood University | 88% |
| MCPHS University, Boston | 95% |
| MCPHS University, Manchester | 93% |
| MCPHS University, Worcester | 93% |
| Medical University of South Carolina | 96% |
| Mercer University | 94% |
| Mercy College | 87% |
| Mercyhurst University | TBD |
| Methodist University | 97% |
| MGH Institute of Health Professions | TBD |
| Miami-Dade College | 82% |
| Midwestern University, Downers Grove | 98% |
| Midwestern University, Glendale | 98% |
| Misericordia University | 80% (2014–2015) |
| Mississippi College | 93% (2013–2015) |
| Missouri State University | 92% |
| Monmouth University | TBD |
| Mount Saint Mary College | TBD |
| Mount St. Joseph University | TBD |

*(Continued)*

| PA Program | First-Time Pass/Fail Rates |
| --- | --- |
| New York Institute of Technology | 93% |
| Northeastern State University, Oklahoma | TBD |
| Northeastern University | 97% |
| Northern Arizona University | 96% (2014–2015) |
| Northwestern University | 97% (2012–2015) |
| Nova Southeastern University, Fort Lauderdale | 98% |
| Nova Southeastern University, Fort Myers | 94% |
| Nova Southeastern University, Jacksonville | 89% |
| Nova Southeastern University, Orlando | 99% |
| Ohio Dominican University | 98% (2014–2015) |
| Ohio University | TBD |
| Oklahoma City University | TBD |
| Oregon Health & Science University | 98% |
| Our Lady of the Lake College | 87% |
| Pace University | 98% |
| Pacific University | 97% |
| Penn State University | TBD |
| Pennsylvania College of Technology | 87% |
| Philadelphia College of Osteopathic Medicine | 98% |
| Philadelphia University | 94% |
| Quinnipiac University | 98% |
| Red Rocks Community College | 94% |
| Rochester Institute of Technology | 95% |

(Continued)

| PA Program | First-Time Pass/Fail Rates |
| --- | --- |
| Rocky Mountain College | 97% |
| Rocky Mountain University of Health Professions | 86% (2011–2013) |
| Rosalind Franklin University of Medicine | 95% (2012) |
| Rush University | 100% (2013–2016) |
| Rutgers University | 97% |
| Sacred Heart University | TBD |
| Saint Catherine University | 98% (2014–2015) |
| Saint Francis University | 96% |
| Saint Louis University | 99% |
| Salus University | 93% |
| Samuel Merritt University | 92% (2013–2014) |
| Seton Hall University | 99% |
| Seton Hill University | 96% |
| Shenandoah University | 100% (9 yr.) |
| Slippery Rock University | TBD |
| South College | 93% |
| South University | TBD |
| South University, Tampa | 88% (2012–2015) |
| South University, West Palm Beach | TBD |
| Southern California University of Health Sciences | TBD |
| Southern Illinois University | 99% |
| Springfield College | 100% |
| St. Ambrose University | TBD |

(Continued)

| PA Program | First-Time Pass/Fail Rates |
|---|---|
| St. John's University | 86% |
| Stanford University | 90% |
| Stephens College | TBD |
| Stony Brook University | 97% |
| Sullivan University | TBD |
| SUNY Downstate Medical Center | 90% |
| SUNY Upstate Medical Center | 91% |
| Temple University | TBD |
| Texas Tech University Health Sciences Center | 98% |
| Thomas Jefferson University | TBD |
| Touro College, Bay Shore | 97% |
| Touro College, Manhattan | 93% |
| Touro University, California | 98% |
| Touro University Nevada | 93% |
| Towson University CCBC, Essex | 94% |
| Trevecca Nazarene University | 94% |
| Trine University | 93% |
| Tufts University School of Medicine | 100% (2015–2016) |
| Union College | 89% |
| University of Alabama at Birmingham | 97% |
| University of Arkansas | 92% (2015) |
| University of Bridgeport | 88% (2013–2016) |
| University of California-Davis | 97% |

(Continued)

| PA Program | First-Time Pass/Fail Rates |
|---|---|
| University of Charleston | 89% (2015) |
| University of Colorado | 98% |
| University of Dayton | TBD |
| University of Detroit/Mercy | 97% |
| University of Dubuque | TBD |
| University of Evansville | TBD |
| University of Findlay | 92% |
| University of Florida | 99% |
| University of Incarnate Word | TBD |
| University of Iowa | 100% |
| University of Kentucky | 89% |
| University of Maryland Eastern Shore | 86% (2011–2015) |
| University of Missouri, Kansas City | TBD |
| University of Mount Union | 96% |
| University of Nebraska | 98% |
| University of Nevada School of Medicine | TBD |
| University of New England | 94% |
| University of New Mexico | 91% |
| University of North Carolina | TBD |
| University of North Dakota | 89% |
| University of North Texas HS Center Ft Worth | 98% |
| University of Oklahoma, Oklahoma City | 97% |
| University of Oklahoma, Tulsa | 100% (2012–2014) |

*(Continued)*

| PA Program | First-Time Pass/Fail Rates |
|---|---|
| University of Pittsburgh | 92% |
| University of Saint Francis, Fort Wayne | 100% |
| University of South Alabama | 92% |
| University of South Dakota | 90% |
| University of South Florida | TBD |
| University of Southern California | 96% |
| University of St. Francis | 96% |
| University of Tennessee Health Science Center | 92% (2015) |
| University of Texas, HS Center at San Antonio | 95% |
| University of Texas, Medical Branch at Galveston | 98% |
| University of Texas, Pan American | 77% |
| UT Southwestern | 100% |
| University of the Pacific | 97% |
| University of the Sciences of Philadelphia | TBD |
| University of Toledo | 95% |
| University of Utah | 93% |
| University of Washington | 86% |
| University of Wisconsin, La Crosse | 100% |
| University of Wisconsin, Madison | 97% |
| Wagner College | 96% |
| Wake Forest University | 97% |
| Wayne State University | 96% |

*(Continued)*

| PA Program | First-Time Pass/Fail Rates |
|---|---|
| West Liberty University | 94% (2014–2015) |
| Western Michigan University | 91% |
| Western University of Health Sciences | 90% |
| Wichita State University | 96% |
| Wingate University | 96% |
| Yale University School of Medicine | 98% |

# PA Programs Utilizing Rolling Admissions (2016)

| PA Program | Rolling Admissions | State |
|---|---|---|
| Adventist University of Health Sciences | NO | FL |
| Albany Medical College | YES | NY |
| Alderson-Broaddus University | YES | WV |
| Anne Arundel Community College | NO | MD |
| Arcadia University | YES | DE/PA |
| Arizona School of Health Sciences | YES | AZ |
| Augsburg College | NO | MN |
| Baldwin Wallace University | NO | OH |
| Barry University | YES | FL |
| Bay Path University | Did Not Respond | MA |
| Baylor College of Medicine | NO | TX |

(*Continued*)

| PA Program | Rolling Admissions | State |
| --- | --- | --- |
| Bethel University | NO | TN |
| Bethel University | NO | MN |
| Boston University | NO | MA |
| Bryant University | YES | RI |
| Butler University | NO | IN |
| Campbell University | YES | NC |
| Carroll University | NO ("pooled") | WI |
| Case Western Reserve University | NO | OH |
| CCNY Sophie Davis School of Biomedical Education | Did Not Respond | NY |
| Central Michigan University | NO | MI |
| Chapman University | Developing | CA |
| Charles R. Drew University | Developing | CA |
| Chatham University | YES | PA |
| Christian Brothers University | NO | TN |
| Clarkson University | YES | NY |
| College of Saint Joseph | Developing | VT |
| College of Saint Scholastica | Developing | MN |
| Concordia University | NO | WI |
| Cornell University | Did Not Respond | NY |
| CUNY York College | NO | NY |
| Cuyahoga Community College/ Cleveland State University | NO | OH |
| D'Youville College | YES | NY |
| Daemen College | NO | NY |

(Continued)

| PA Program | Rolling Admissions | State |
|---|---|---|
| Des Moines University | YES | IA |
| DeSales University | YES | PA |
| Dominican University | Developing (YES) | IL |
| Dominican University of California | Developing | CA |
| Drexel University | YES | PA |
| Duke University Medical Center | YES | NC |
| Duquesne University | YES | PA |
| East Carolina University | YES | NC |
| Eastern Michigan University | NO | MI |
| Eastern Virginia Medical School | NO | VA |
| Elon University | YES | NC |
| Emory University | YES | NC |
| Florida International University Herbert Wertheim College of Medicine | YES | FL |
| Francis Marion University | Developing (NO) | SC |
| Franklin College | Developing | IN |
| Franklin Pierce University | NO | NH |
| Gannon University | NO | PA |
| Gardner Webb University | YES | NC |
| George Washington University | NO | DC |
| Georgia Regents University | YES | GA |
| Grand Valley State University | Did Not Respond | MI |
| Hardin-Simmons University | Developing (YES) | TX |
| Harding University | YES | AK |

(Continued)

| PA Program | Rolling Admissions | State |
|---|---|---|
| Heritage University | YES | WA |
| High Point University | YES | NC |
| Hofstra University | YES | NY |
| Howard University | Did Not Respond | DC |
| Idaho State University | NO | ID |
| Indiana State University | Did Not Respond | IN |
| Indiana Univ. School of Health and Rehab. Sciences | NO | IN |
| Interservice | Military Only | |
| James Madison University | YES | VA |
| Jefferson College of Health Sciences | YES | VA |
| Johnson & Wales University | YES | RI |
| Kean University | Developing | NJ |
| Keiser University | YES | FL |
| Kettering College | "Somewhat" | OH |
| King's College | NO | PA |
| Lake Erie College | YES | OH |
| Le Moyne College | NO | NY |
| Lenoir-Rhyne University | YES | NC |
| Lincoln Memorial | YES | TN |
| Lock Haven University | NO | PA |
| Loma Linda University | NO | CA |
| Long Island University | NO | NY |
| Louisiana State University, New Orleans | NO | LA |

*(Continued)*

| PA Program | Rolling Admissions | State |
|---|---|---|
| Louisiana State University, Shreveport | ("Quasi") | LA |
| Lynchburg College | YES | VA |
| Marietta College | YES | OH |
| Marist College | YES | NY |
| Marquette University | Did Not Respond | WI |
| Marshall B. Ketchum University | NO | CA |
| Mary Baldwin College | YES | VA |
| Marywood University | Did Not Respond | PA |
| MCPHS University, Boston | YES | MA |
| MCPHS University, Manchester | YES | NH |
| MCPHS University, Worcester | YES | MA |
| Medical University of South Carolina | NO | SC |
| Mercer University | YES | GA |
| Mercy College | Did Not Respond | NY |
| Mercyhurst University | NO | PA |
| Methodist University | YES | NC |
| MGH Institute of Health Professions | NO | MA |
| Miami-Dade College | Did Not Respond | FL |
| Midwestern University, Downers Grove | YES | IL |
| Midwestern University, Glendale | YES | AZ |
| Misericordia University | YES | PA |
| Mississippi College | YES | MS |

*(Continued)*

| PA Program | Rolling Admissions | State |
|---|---|---|
| Missouri State University | NO | MO |
| Monmouth University | YES | NJ |
| Mount Saint Mary College | Developing | NY |
| Mount St. Joseph University | Developing | OH |
| New York Institute of Technology | NO | NY |
| Northeastern State University, Oklahoma | NO | OK |
| Northeastern University | NO | MA |
| Northern Arizona University | NO | AZ |
| Northwestern University | YES | IL |
| Nova Southeastern University, Fort Lauderdale | YES | FL |
| Nova Southeastern University, Fort Myers | YES | FL |
| Nova Southeastern University, Jacksonville | YES | FL |
| Nova Southeastern University, Orlando | YES | FL |
| Ohio Dominican University | YES | OH |
| Ohio University | NO | OH |
| Oklahoma City University | NO | OK |
| Oregon Health & Science University | YES | OR |
| Our Lady of the Lake College | YES | LA` |
| Pace University | NO | NY |
| Pacific University | NO | OR |

*(Continued)*

| PA Program | Rolling Admissions | State |
|---|---|---|
| Penn State University | Did Not Respond | PA |
| Pennsylvania College of Technology | NO | PA |
| Philadelphia College of Osteopathic Medicine | YES | PA |
| Philadelphia University | YES | PA |
| Quinnipiac University | NO | CT |
| Red Rocks Community College | NO | CO |
| Rochester Institute of Technology | NO | NY |
| Rocky Mountain College | YES | MT |
| Rocky Mountain University of Health Professions | NO | UT |
| Rosalind Franklin University of Medicine | YES | IL |
| Rush University | YES | IL |
| Rutgers University | YES | NJ |
| Sacred Heart University | Developing (NO) | CT |
| Saint Catherine University | NO | MN |
| Saint Francis University | YES | PA |
| Saint Louis University | Modified | MO |
| Salus University | YES | PA |
| Samuel Merritt University | YES | CA |
| Seton Hall University | Did Not Respond | NJ |
| Seton Hill University | NO | PA |
| Shenandoah University | YES | VA |

(Continued)

| PA Program | Rolling Admissions | State |
| --- | --- | --- |
| Slippery Rock University | Developing | PA |
| South College | YES | TN |
| South University | Did Not Respond | GA |
| South University, Tampa | NO | FL |
| South University, West Palm Beach | Developing | FL |
| Southern California University of Health Sciences | Developing (NO) | CA |
| Southern Illinois University | YES | IL |
| Springfield College | YES | MA |
| St. Ambrose University | NO | IA |
| St. John's University | NO | NY |
| Stanford University | NO | CA |
| Stephens College | Developing | MO |
| Stony Brook University | YES | NY |
| Sullivan University | NO | KY |
| SUNY Downstate Medical Center | NO | NY |
| SUNY Upstate Medical Center | NO | NY |
| Temple University | Developing | PA |
| Texas Tech University Health Sciences Center | YES | TX |
| Thomas Jefferson University | YES | PA |
| Touro College, Bay Shore | NO | NY |
| Touro College, Manhattan | YES | NY |
| Touro University, California | YES | CA |

(Continued)

| PA Program | Rolling Admissions | State |
|---|---|---|
| Touro University Nevada | YES | NV |
| Towson University CCBC, Essex | YES | MD |
| Trevecca Nazarene University | NO | TN |
| Trine University | Developing | IN |
| Tufts University School of Medicine | YES | MA |
| Union College | NO | NE |
| University of Alabama at Birmingham | NO | AL |
| University of Arkansas | Did Not Respond | AK |
| University of Bridgeport | NO | CT |
| University of California-Davis | NO | CA |
| University of Charleston | NO | WV |
| University of Colorado | YES | CO |
| University of Dayton | NO | OH |
| University of Detroit/Mercy | NO | MI |
| University of Dubuque | Developing | IA |
| University of Evansville | Developing | IN |
| University of Findlay | NO | OH |
| University of Florida | NO | FL |
| University of Incarnate Word | Developing | TX |
| University of Iowa | YES | IA |
| University of Kentucky | NO | KY |
| University of Maryland Eastern Shore | Did Not Respond | MD |

(Continued)

| PA Program | Rolling Admissions | State |
|---|---|---|
| University of Missouri, Kansas City | NO | MO |
| University of Mount Union | NO | OH |
| University of Nebraska | NO | NE |
| University of Nevada School of Medicine | Developing | NV |
| University of New England | YES | ME |
| University of New Mexico | NO | NM |
| University of North Carolina | NO | NC |
| University of North Dakota | NO | ND |
| University of North Texas HS Center Ft Worth | YES | TX |
| University Of Oklahoma, Oklahoma City | NO | OK |
| University of Oklahoma, Tulsa | NO | OK |
| University of Pittsburgh | YES | PA |
| University of Saint Francis, Fort Wayne | YES | IN |
| University of South Alabama | Did Not Respond | AL |
| University of South Dakota | NO | SD |
| University of South Florida | Developing | FL |
| University of Southern California | YES | CA |
| University of St. Francis | YES | NM |
| University of Tennessee Health Science Center | Did Not Respond | TN |
| University of Texas HS Center at San Antonio | YES | TX |

(Continued)

| PA Program | Rolling Admissions | State |
|---|---|---|
| University of Texas, Medical Branch at Galveston | NO | TX |
| University of Texas, Pan American | YES | TX |
| UT Southwestern | NO | TX |
| University of the Pacific | Developing (YES) | CA |
| University of the Sciences of Philadelphia | YES | PA |
| University of Toledo | NO | OH |
| University of Utah | NO | UT |
| University of Washington | YES | WA |
| University of Wisconsin, La Crosse | NO | WI |
| University of Wisconsin, Madison | NO | WI |
| Wagner College | NO | NY |
| Wake Forest University | YES | NC |
| Wayne State University | NO | MI |
| West Liberty University | YES | WV |
| Western Michigan University | YES | MI |
| Western University of Health Sciences | Did Not Respond | CA |
| Wichita State University | NO | KS |
| Wingate University | YES | NC |
| Yale University School of Medicine | YES | CT |

# APPENDIX 5

# Writing an Effective Letter of Recommendation

The purpose of the letter of recommendation (LOR) is to provide the admissions committee with a detailed description of an applicant's abilities and qualities, rather than to merely check off a box on the CASPA application.

Let's take a look at a sample LOR, then dissect it and point out the three key elements that make a great LOR.

Dear Ms. Dean:

Please accept this correspondence a strong recommendation for John Smith's application as a student in your physician assistant program. I am the current Dean of the College of Health and Human Performance at Mankato State University, and John was my student for 4 years and my teaching assistant for 2 years.

As a student, John was easily in the top 10% of his peers for 4 years in a row. John is intelligent, energetic, reliable, and above all he is a team player.

As my teaching assistant, John was rated the highest by more than 122 students who have taken my classes. He scored high in communication skills, knowledge base, and likeability. He proved himself to be a dedicated, hardworking, and diligent young man.

John also has a strong military background. He served for 4 years as a navy corpsman, and his experience in that position would provide great strength to his candidacy in your PA program, and as a PA in the future. He was also an air force officer, which explains his admirable ability to pay strict attention to detail.

This young man has a high social conscience, high energy, a cooperative style, and the uncanny ability to analyze complex problems in the health field in simple yet constructive context. His social graces are beyond reproach. John will make an outstanding PA. He really cares for people, and people care for him.

I strongly recommend John Smith for candidacy in your physician assistant program.

Sincerely,

Robert R. Rockingham, Ph.D.
Dean, College of Health and Human Performance
Mankato State University

## CONTENT

This LOR contains three key elements of an appropriate and effective letter of recommendation:

1. Introduction and background of the writer
2. Writer's relationship to the candidate
3. Quantified claims rather than general statements

The purpose of the writer introducing himself in the opening paragraph is to qualify as a legitimate reference. It shows that the reference truly knows the applicant and can honestly and objectively comment on the applicant's achievements, interpersonal and organizational skills, communication skills, and so on.

Finally, the reference quantifies the applicant's claims. Many people make it seem like they can walk on water in their applications. If the writer uses "meaningful specifics" versus "wandering generalities," he or she lends more credence to the letter (e.g., "was rated highest by more than 122 students").

## IDENTIFY CANDIDATE'S STRENGTHS

A powerful LOR does not simply recite the obvious: "Sue has a great GPA." It's quite obvious to the committee that Sue has a 3.7 GPA; it's on her CASPA application.

The writer should be more creative and spend enough time on the letter to make you stand out from the crowd. The writer is usually asked to evaluate the applicant in several areas:

- Academic performance
- Interpersonal skills
- Maturity
- Adaptability and flexibility
- Motivation for a career as a PA

The writer may comment on all of these areas or just a few. In the areas that the writer does choose to comment on, his/her comments should be specific and relevant to that area.

For instance:

- Academic performance: "Top 10% of his peers."
- Interpersonal skills: "He cares for people, and people care for him."
- Maturity: "A strong military background."
- Adaptability and flexibility: "The uncanny ability to analyze complex problems...in simple yet constructive terms."

## FINAL THOUGHTS

1. Go back to the sample letter and highlight all of the qualities about John that are mentioned. Remember, "it's not about you, it's about them." The committee already knows the qualities that they are seeking in the perfect applicant and the more qualities that are mentioned in the LOR, the better fit you will be for the program.

2. It is very important to keep the letter short, concise, specific, and personal. If someone else's name can be substituted for yours without changing the content of the letter, it is too generic.

3. Be sure the writer is recommending you for PA school and not Medical School.

# Sample Essays

## ESSAY 1: CHILDHOOD/FAMILY EXPERIENCES

"One time, a family cat captured...a moth. The cat's play disturbed E., who promptly got a local veterinarian on the phone to get tips on reviving the mortally wounded moth. The moth didn't make it, but knowing E.'s enthusiasm, Mrs. E. is more optimistic about the park." (The Idaho Statesman, November 22, 1978)

This article, about me as a 10-year-old boy trying to turn a nearby drainage pond into a park, had a misprint—it was a mouse, not a moth. Still, this example shows why people have always said I would probably be a doctor or veterinarian. Wandering the fields, I brought home sick and hurt creatures; if anyone found an injured bird or animal, they brought it to me for care.

We didn't exactly live on a farm, but were in farming country. My father always made sure that we had a large garden; that, along with a small vineyard, orchard, and corn field, provided work for us six kids and a little extra family income. My parents couldn't give us allowances and we had to help pay for our own clothes, so we worked on local farms (bucking hay bales, moving sprinkler pipes, etc.) and did whatever we could find—I started an early morning daily paper route (on my bike, in all weather) at age 11, and had it for 5 years.

During this period, we did manage to find time for other things. Besides earning the rank of Eagle Scout, I sang in school choirs, performed in state piano boards, acted in school and community theater, ran (and earned a letter) in cross-country and track (until forced by my Junior year to choose between school sports and earning money), and served as a student body representative in my high school.

After two semesters at Boise State, I volunteered to serve for 2 years as a missionary with the Church of Jesus Christ of Latter-Day Saints, going to the California, Ventura Mission. I loved it, learned a lot, being able to dedicate every hour to helping and teaching people of all nationalities, cultures, and religions. Many of the friends I made among the people and the other missionaries are still very close, and the lessons I learned from all of my experiences affect my life every day.

Returning to school, my classes included math and sciences (subjects' I had shied away from before)—out of curiosity, at first; then, to keep my options open. I actually enjoyed them, and managed to get good grades. My love for the humanities continued, including writing guest editorials and articles for the Fullerton College school paper, and I was awarded the annual Book Award for Excellence in Foreign Language from the Spanish department. My activities were rounded out by helping at a nearby adolescent rehabilitation clinic, and serving the single members of my church as the activities committee chairman and representative to the regional council.

In high school, I had some health problems and seen a number of doctors. When a general practitioner didn't find anything, he sent me to a specialist, who sent me to another, who sent me to another...none of whom could find a problem, yet all of whom charged my parents what seemed exorbitant fees.

This experience soured me on the medical profession. My interests in people continued to grow, but because of my cynicism toward physicians and lack of money, medical school wasn't seriously considered. Besides, math and sciences didn't appeal to me at that time like music, drama, philosophy, and writing did.

I pursued psychology and the humanities, while growing more fascinated by health, nutrition, and what people I knew had found in "alternative" approaches to health, including preventive and Eastern medicine. Although a natural skeptic, it seemed to me that if something appears to work for rational, respectable people, it should be taken seriously—researched, to determine whether the benefit is merely psychological or not—contrary to the doctors I had met, who felt that if THEY didn't have it, it was "dangerous." This seemed narrow-minded, opposing the principles I understood "science" to be based upon.

Upon transferring to USC, I found that my view of the medical establishment wasn't really accurate—there ARE those who care more about helping people than about the money or their intellectual pride. As a result,

I've decided to enter medical school, focusing on research and preventive medicine. My major in Exercise Science is providing a strong background in physiology and nutrition.

Throughout my college career, I have had to support myself financially. Working full-time while at Boise State as a restaurant manager, and then doing singing telegrams, fitness consulting, and running my own window-cleaning business since moving to California have allowed me to get by. Now, my work-study research job at the LA County General Hospital/USC Health Sciences Campus is also providing excellent experience in working in both hospital and research settings. My church responsibilities continually mean opportunities for volunteer service, and as Vice-President of the USC chapter of S. fraternity, one of my projects has been setting up and directing our relationship with Challengers, a local inner-city youth club with which our fraternity is now involved in activities and tutoring.

# ESSAY 2: WOMEN'S CLINIC VOLUNTEER

It was opening night. I was about to walk on stage as Ruth in "The Pirates of Penzance." Any sane actor would be singing scales, or meditating, or reviewing dialogue. I was spitting into a test tube. Later, I would assay the saliva for cortisol and compare the results with my normal cortisol levels. Discovering what was happening in my body as the curtain prepared to rise was worth the temporary distraction from the pirate king.

"Spit happens," as we say in my lab. Spit happened to me during the summer after my sophomore year in college. I worked in the Reproductive Ecology Laboratory at Harvard University, measuring steroid hormones in saliva by radioimmunoassay. I had never considered myself a science whiz, and I took the job with a little trepidation. I pipetted until my thumb ached and washed an endless stream of glassware, but the end result was something amazing. With those tiny vials of saliva, I could track my menstrual cycle. I could measure my brother's testosterone levels, or my own—which I hadn't even known I had. I realized that I was doing science. I was doing it well and enjoying it. I went on to complete my senior honors thesis on the relationship between cortisol levels and temperament in shy adolescents. In the lab, I discovered the fascination of research and the discipline needed to carry it out. I am excited to be continuing my work there as a researcher and teaching assistant for the 1993 to 1994 school year.

About the same time spit happened to me, I found myself writing research papers on a consistent set of themes. For my women's history class, I wrote about the turn of the century movement for "twilight sleep" anesthesia in childbirth. For my sophomore tutorial in anthropology, I researched the effects of social support on the duration and complications of labor and delivery. For my sociology class, I investigated the controversy surrounding the Depo Provera contraceptive. My passion for these topics and my interest in science fueled a growing desire to go to medical school. I began taking premed classes and continued pursuing these interests, both in and out of the classroom.

At Lutheran General Hospital in Park Ridge, Illinois, I studied patients who had undergone laparoscopic surgery for uterine fibroids and ovarian cysts. While gathering clinical data, reading literature, and observing surgeries, I was amazed by the results of such noninvasive techniques, and had visions of holding the laparoscope myself in a few years. I enjoyed being part of the rhythms of a busy obstetrics and gynecology practice and solidified my desire to be a doctor.

As a volunteer in a women's health clinic in Boston, during my senior year in college, I answered phones and made appointments and referrals. I discovered how much good I could do just by listening and focusing my attention on the person on the phone. That simple act did so much to alleviate a woman's worries and uncertainties. I also learned to treat each patient with fairness and decency, regardless of her circumstances. I know that the things I can accomplish listening with the additional skills of a physician are extraordinary.

Much of my remaining spare time in college was spent working in theater. While president of the Harvard-Radcliffe Gilbert and Sullivan Players, I led a board of 15 strong-willed, outspoken peers. I made sure each person was heard in discussions and that the group remained focused. As producer of several plays, I was thrilled to watch the curtain rise, knowing I had harnessed the energies and talents of dozens of people to make the show happen. Through my work in theater, I learned to keep my stress levels reasonable and my temper intact while juggling innumerable tasks—usually on very few hours of sleep.

In college, I became one-part scientist, one-part counselor, and one-part leader. My interest in how our bodies work and how we relate to those bodies continues to grow in tandem with my vision of myself as a physician. I know that with the skills I gained in college, from techniques in the laboratory to group leadership in theater production to listening and compassion on the clinic telephone, I am well prepared to enter medical school. And I can't wait to see what it does to my cortisol levels.

## Student Comments

"As I recall, it took me between 6 and 8 weeks to write this essay, including time to mail it back and forth to my premed advisor for critiquing. In the original version, I fantasized about being trapped in an elevator with a pregnant woman and delivering her baby while we waited for the repairmen. My advisor felt that scenario was too frivolous and silly sounding, so I changed it to the (true) story that starts this version."

# ESSAY 3: HOSPITAL VOLUNTEER

As the rusted-out Land Rover made its way cautiously through dense thicket and crevices in the rocky dirt road, those of us sitting on top were able to peer through the trees at a sublime West African landscape. Our destination was S., a tiny village 300 miles upcountry where running water and electricity were unheard of...let alone access to basic health care. This was the summer of my freshman year at Brown, when I joined a multinational team on a medical development project in Sierra Leone. One afternoon a woman who had trekked many miles through the jungle to find care approached our clinic with an infant in her arms. She was not lactating effectively, and her child lay emaciated and dying. As I held the baby and administered a simple oral rehydration therapy and taught the mother to do the same, I was overcome with the sense of my relationship to this child and mother and by my ability to make a tangible difference in people's lives through the act of healing—the essence of being a physician.

My desire to become a doctor has developed through several years of academic, professional, and volunteer work as well as personal introspection. These have strengthened my conviction that through medicine I will be able to make a meaningful contribution to people's lives on both the individual and societal levels. Moreover, I hope that my various experiences will help me to be a broader, more informed, and more sensitive physician.

Reflecting on my endeavors, I see a common theme of humanitarian concern—a sensibility that grew out of early experiences living abroad with my family. As I became acquainted with myriad cultures, I developed an appreciation for the similarities and differences between societies. But more profoundly, witnessing vast basic needs in developing countries shaped my resolve to make a difference by serving others. Early on I looked to medicine as a means of doing so, and during high school I volunteered in a renal research lab. Joining daily rounds and visiting patients who would benefit from the research gave meaning to the work. I was also inspired by the positive impact that my father, a physician, had on people's lives.

At Brown and Oxford my interests in culture and in the difficulties of cross-cultural communication drew me to study the relationships between literature, society, and politics. I discovered literature's unique ability to articulate the human connections that underlie cultural differences: this provided an intellectual underpinning for my commitment to public service, particularly for my involvement in campus race relations issues. In addition, my studies of the sociopolitical components of underdevelopment taught me that improved infrastructure and health education might have prevented many of the conditions we had treated in Africa. I acted on my growing policy concerns by working with the U.S. State Department in Nigeria and at the B. Institution, where I gained firsthand insight into policy formulation.

But I soon realized that helping people in a direct and tangible way held greater meaning for me than did the arena of policy. When thinking seriously about a career path, my early interests in medicine were renewed as I reflected on how fulfilling my volunteer experiences had been, particularly working with patients in Sierra Leone and in a hospital context. I had also been inspired in Nigeria, seeing the contribution dedicated physicians made to the quality of people's lives in poor areas—and the acute need for doctors in underserved regions. And I recognized that within the field of health care policy, the input of experienced physicians is vital when designing programs. Acting on this decision, I served as an emergency room volunteer in Washington and applied to the Bryn Mawr Post Baccalaureate Program. At Bryn Mawr I have been struck by my flourishing interest in the scientific side of medicine, particularly molecular genetics, oncology, and neurology. I have followed my clinical interests by volunteering at Hahnemann. This spring I will be returning to Sierra Leone with a grassroots medical development organization to work setting up rural health clinics and to write a report outlining regional health care priorities.

A separate part of my life, my love for and involvement with music, has enhanced my appreciation for creativity and for the discipline of fine tuning a skill. An especially rewarding quality of music is the way it can forge connections between people: while touring Spain with a jazz ensemble we encountered a group of children with Down's syndrome. At first they seemed detached, but when we played for them they became animated—dancing, laughing, and smiling. Such experiences have impressed on me that relating to people is a vital component of healing.

This past year at Bryn Mawr has confirmed for me that medicine is a dynamic field in which I can bring together my interests in development policy and in serving people directly as a physician. I believe that the skills I have acquired through research, the study of literature, policy analysis, volunteer work, music, and cross-cultural interaction will continue to develop within medicine and will enable me to make a meaningful contribution.

## ESSAY 4: HIGH SCHOOL HOSPITAL VOLUNTEER

Dr. Lewis Thomas described medicine as "The Youngest Science" because insightful discoveries in basic research have led to revolutionary innovations in clinical therapy that have improved the quality of life. We are in the midst of an exciting era in which our knowledge about the molecular aspects of medicine is growing each day. I feel that the medical profession uniquely integrates my passion for science with my desire to work with others. Medicine is boundless; like no other profession, it wholly captures my intellectual ideals and humanistic values.

I have been curious about medicine since childhood. To learn about the profession, I would pose questions to the physicians in my own family. Eager to gain hands-on experience, I volunteered in high school at the St. Joseph's Hospital in [hometown]. I had the opportunity to escort patients from one area of the hospital to another prior to diagnostic tests or treatments. Through interactions with many patients, I discovered the therapeutic and comforting effects of an encouraging smile and a friendly conversation. From observing patients with simple correctable problems, such as a hernia, to those with chronic problems, such as rheumatoid arthritis, I gained an understanding for a physician's daily challenges.

Each patient presented a complex array of symptoms that required specialized attention. In order for a physician to help a patient cope with an illness, it was important for him to consider the patient's emotional needs. Especially in stressful situations, I appreciated how the reassuring confidence and warmth, conveyed through a physician's bedside manner, gradually transformed a patient's immediate fears into strength and hope.

Medicine offers diverse opportunities to interact with others. In the past, I have found service-oriented activities to be particularly rewarding. In high school, I felt that I could most effectively contribute to my local community by participating in student government. As Student Council President, I interacted with individuals with a variety of personalities to ensure that my peers had the opportunity to express their ideas and opinions freely. At XXXXXX University, I discovered that the most vital component of campus life was living in the residence hall. Therefore, after my freshman year, I decided to become a Resident Advisor (RA). One of my personal goals was to encourage each resident to take full advantage of our unique living situation. As a diverse community, we had many experiences to share with each other. I enjoyed organizing activities such as discussions, educational programs, and study breaks that helped form an interactive and supportive community. For the past 2 years, some of my most rewarding experiences have emerged from my dynamic role as a peer counselor and resource figure. One of the most challenging situations that I encountered was when our floor custodian informed me about the packaged bags of regurgitated food that he found in the women's bathroom over several weeks. By consulting fellow staff members and recruiting the help of health professionals, my co-RA and I organized educational programs about eating disorders to address this sensitive situation. Fortunately, there were no further occurrences. By helping my peers cope with the stresses of college life as an RA, I not only gained valuable interpersonal skills, but also formed lasting friendships.

Another interest that I have explored is my fascination with the creative and unpredictable diversity of living organisms. With a fervent interest in biology, I joined the genetics laboratory of Dr. X. in my freshman year. After learning about the biology of the ciliated protozoan, *Tetrahymena thermophila*, I focused my efforts on understanding the mechanism of strain-specific, age-dependent micronuclear degradation. With the support of the Howard Hughes Scholar Program for Undergraduates, I cloned transposon-like elements in *Tetrahymena* that may cause chromosomal rearrangements associated with age-dependent micronuclear degradation. The multitude of puzzles that I encountered in the laboratory challenged my creativity and fostered intellectual development that I could not attain in a classroom. By critically analyzing experimental obstacles, I gained invaluable problem-solving skills. In my senior year, I will further investigate this intriguing model of aging as part of my honors thesis.

Because my research experience has added a unique dimension to my education, I feel that it is important to support the research interests of others. As an executive board member of the X. Undergraduate Research Board, I have assisted students in finding faculty members with similar research interests. This past year, I took part in organizing a forum for students to present their research findings to the Cornell community.

This summer, I have engaged in an internship that has enhanced my understanding of the relationship between basic research and medicine. By working with Dr. X. at the Memorial Sloan-Kettering Cancer Center, I discovered the excitement that surrounds the emerging science and technology that will lead to future innovations in medicine. A long-term goal of Dr. X's laboratory is to develop retroviral-mediated gene therapy for patients with chronic hemolytic anemia due to a severe deficiency of glucose-6-phosphate dehydrogenase (G6PD). I tested the efficiency of replication-defective retroviral vectors that are capable of transferring the human G6PD gene to cells in vitro. The existence of inherited diseases such as severe G6PD deficiency, cystic fibrosis, adenosine deaminase deficiency, and others that are clinically manageable, but incurable, presents a unique problem to the medical community. Ideally, I wish to be involved in both the traditional primary care of these patients and investigative research that may lead to more effective therapy.

I aspire to become a physician because to me, it is the world's most vibrant and rewarding profession. The practice of medicine offers a daily sense of fulfillment that is rare. Basic and clinical research enhances our understanding of disease and provides us with the tools to improve the lives of many. As a lifelong commitment to society, the medical profession most completely encompasses my career goals and moral values.

## ESSAY 5: MOTIVATED BY CHILDHOOD ILLNESS

My work experiences—ranging from public health projects in rural Latin America to work at urban battered women's shelters to peer counseling on a college campus—reflect my concern for people's "health" in a broad sense of the word. Yet I never imagined as an undergraduate in the social sciences that I would eventually become a doctor. I also never expected to call rehydration salts "anti-witch" treatment, but suddenly, one day, that made perfect sense.

The morning of New Year's Day, 1978, was bright and sunny. Refreshed from a good night's sleep, I lifted the blankets, rose to my feet, and collapsed, unable to walk. Soon afterwards, emergency room doctors assured me that it was only a temporary viral infection and not, as my parents worried, a handicapping case of polio. I recovered from that frightening infection, but imprinted in my mind is the feeling of relief I felt at the hospital, where I could be confident about the professionals looking after me. This experience prompted me to consider dedicating my life to becoming a doctor, helping others, and giving them the same confidence I felt in that emergency room. Caring for my arthritis-afflicted mother for the past several years and volunteering at a local hospital have helped me realize that I have the compassion that motivates me to become a medical professional.

Despite having various interests, I have carefully determined to pursue an MD-PhD program. My experiences have led me to believe that I will make an effective clinical physician since I enjoy working with people one-on-one, but that my other talents can be used to make even more far-reaching contributions to medicine and to society. As a newsroom teleprompter operator, I have been exposed to broadcasting and realize that I would enjoy delivering reports as a medical correspondent. I see the need for qualified medical personnel in the media to function as interpreters of medical knowledge for the general public. Though this is an option, my experiences in research have helped me decide to seek a career primarily as a scientific investigator.

My transcript and various awards, which include the UW Dean's Medal for the Sciences, demonstrate my academic ability, but research has been the most satisfying component of my undergraduate education. It has allowed me to develop my intellectual curiosity by applying learned knowledge to new situations. For the last 2 years, I have been characterizing particular site-specific mutations in the envelope glycoprotein of the human immunodeficiency virus (HIV) under the supervision of Dr. S. My planning and performing of experiments, collection of results, and conducting of extensive literature searches were brought together into a cohesive whole as my honors senior thesis, which was selected as the best undergraduate paper in Microbiology and awarded the J. Ordal Award.

The results of my work are presented in a manuscript, which is being submitted for publication. Also, I have contributed to a poster abstract at a recent international AIDS vaccines conference.

Since I would like to practice in both the clinic and the lab and therefore need to be much more than just a technician, I am currently completing a second degree in Speech Communication. Effective communication is crucial in all aspects of our lives, but particularly for physicians, who must be especially sensitive to the needs of their patients in the clinic and must be able to communicate clearly with colleagues as scientists. The opportunities I have had to develop interpersonal and public-speaking skills are directly relevant to helping me become a better clinician and researcher.

Although completing two degrees and working have demanded much time, I have not allowed them to hinder my participation in activities which have helped me mature as a person. Serving as a counselor for junior-high youths in our church, leading bible studies, and operating the closed-circuit camera during Sunday services have given me important lessons about working with people. Studying piano for 12 years and learning tennis as a new sport have taught me the value of perseverance, dedication, and self-discipline. All of these activities, especially doubles tennis, have helped me become a better team player.

Wanting to become a doctor is not a recent desire, but a result of experiences over my lifetime. My willingness to work hard and to persevere through difficult and demanding situations, as well as my ability to relate to others will enhance my capacity to contribute to society as a doctor. Equally important, however, is that I expect to be satisfied as a research and clinical physician, intellectually challenged and content knowing that I am doing my best to help others.

## Student Comments

"This essay actually took me several weeks (on-and-off, of course) of writing. I felt that giving details about how my interest in medicine developed over time would set my essay apart from those of applicants who just simply stated that they wanted to help others. I think the most difficult aspect of the writing process was trying to emphasize what I thought were my strong selling points without bragging, and I believe giving detailed examples helped in this regard."

# ESSAY 6: FAMILY PHYSICIANS, MOTIVATED SINCE CHILDHOOD

Initially, my interest in medicine was due to my family. Several of my relatives are physicians and they have always been enthusiastic about their hospital work. From their discussions on various diseases, I became very curious and disturbed about why all human beings inevitably age and die. I grew up being both impressed with all of the medical treatments available and dismayed by stories of the terminally ill. The human body was repairable but fragile. To be alive and healthy was a fascination.

These childhood impressions were strong ones, and when I began college, I felt deeply intrigued with medicine. During my college years, I studied a good deal of chemistry and biology, and as my interests in various sciences grew, I tried some hospital volunteer work. While pursuing my assorted interests, my captivation with medicine not only endured, but also has remained to be my ultimate interest.

My most direct exposure to medicine was my volunteer work in hospital emergency rooms. The most enjoyable part of my job was taking patients who were on stretchers or in wheelchairs to various areas of the hospital and keeping them company. I enjoyed doing so, and I also found myself wishing that I had the skill and knowledge to examine and treat them. I also noticed how the physicians, nurses, and aides all worked together. I was left with a vivid impression that the hospital was a close-knit team of different professionals, of which I wished to be a part of.

Teaching chemistry has also been a very positive experience. During my sophomore year and junior years, I was a tutor for an accelerated chemistry lab course. Acting on the belief that more help should be available for this rigorous class, I began a tutoring program, which continues to this day. I could relate to the students' frustrations and I held classroom sessions for groups of students ranging from 5 to 25, covering questions dealing with laboratory procedures, reports, and problem sets. After 2 years of tutoring, I felt it would be more challenging to teach a different class and I am presently a teaching assistant for a chemistry lecture course. From these teaching experiences, I have learned to communicate effectively to large groups of people and also to individuals on a one-to-one basis. I have become more sensitive to people's problems and needs and create an environment that encourages discussions and questions. My relationships with the students have been the most gratifying aspect of teaching, and as a physician, I hope to feel the same type of satisfaction from interacting with my patients.

During my summers, I have had an opportunity to work in various research laboratories. In order to sample different areas in science, I worked in labs ranging from inorganic chemistry to molecular biology. In all cases, I learned to conduct experiments in an orderly yet creative manner and I was constantly collecting data and interpreting results. Most importantly, I learned to accept my defeats graciously when my experiments failed. Last summer at M.I.T., I performed many experiments with unsatisfactory results, but I was able to finish my project and I will be the first author of a publication.

By becoming a physician, I will be able to solve medical problems while treating and being in constant contact with patients. Being a physician will be quite demanding and difficult at times, but most of all, I imagine that it will be most enjoyable and quite satisfying.

## Student Comments

"In my essay, I just wrote about things I felt proud of: my family background, volunteer work, teaching, and research. I could have written much more on my research experience but I didn't because I knew that my recommendation letters would include that information in detail. As a personal opinion, I think that as long as the essay is reasonably well written, it's fine.

In terms of medical school admission advice, I tell people that just like in real life, connections are very important and so the letters of recommendation are very crucial. Yes, I had all A's and my MCAT scores were good but I think my letters of recommendation were almost the most important. The people who wrote my letters of recommendation were from University of Illinois or from Harvard and I got into those med schools. So if someone is panicked that he/she won't get into any medical school, they should definitely apply to the schools they have close affiliations with. If all other criteria are good, it's a good chance he/she will get into that school. Many students at Harvard (my classmates right now) also took an extra year to do research work and that also helps greatly in terms of a strong recommendation letter and what kind of an essay you can write by taking extra time off to do research and volunteer work. It is also very much worth the experience."

# ESSAY 7: ROWER

"Power ten, next stoke!" shouts the coxswain over the speaker system. We rush past English countryside as our rowing shell skims along the River Cam. "One—drive it hard! Two! Three!" Each rower in the eight quietly focuses on his own stroke, not communicating with anyone. In the midst of the physical exertion of taking stroke after stroke, I am amazed by what I am doing and where I am doing it.

I chose to go to Cambridge for a year abroad because I thought a year in England would add a new dimension to my education, both culturally and academically. New York is always stimulating, but I wanted to experience life somewhere else. I intuitively knew that a change of perspective would be rewarding. I was determined to continue my scientific studies, and Cambridge offers some of the best academic science in the world. I was excited to have been awarded a place in the university. Happily, I found an activity, which enabled me to both immerse myself in English culture and achieve a sense of personal accomplishment. That activity was rowing.

I chose to row for several reasons. Rowing provided an effective way to meet many people and assimilate into English life. I turned down an offer to join the Cambridge sailing team because I felt that rowing would better introduce me to English culture. Sailing for another year would have been the predictable, safe option; I wanted a new challenge. Rowing was Cambridge's most popular and traditional sport. I was eager to learn new customs and acquire a mastery over a new skill. In addition, disciplined exercise has always helped me to focus on important things in my life, like doing school work or deciding to go to medical school.

Never having rowed before, I had to start from the bottom, in a novice boat. Practice commenced before sunrise, and we had to run down to the boathouse each morning because, as we were told, every rower going back over a hundred years had to do it. We practiced in leaky, old wooden boats that had their heyday back in the 1950s. Yelling commands through dented-in megaphones, 60-year-old coaches dressed in tweed followed us along the bank in bicycles older than they were.

The richness of the English rowing tradition inspired me. The boathouse was strewn with historic championship awards bearing inscriptions from places as far away as communist Russia and as near as prestigious Henley. While my boat did not contribute to the grand collection, I did have the satisfaction of upholding the tradition and high standard of rowing in England by being a participant.

After much improvement, I was promoted to the college's second boat by the second term. The second boat required much more commitment to training. I had never been in so fit and focused before in my life. It was a challenge to maintain such a high level of performance, but my diligence paid dividends as we were placed among the top boats in our regattas.

One of my goals while abroad had been to travel around England, using Cambridge as a starting point for journeys to various towns and cities. My plans were curtailed because rowing required so much of my time, and I was determined to finish what I had started and to see my commitment through. I discovered that rowing on a short stretch of the Cam enriched my education more than any traveling could do.

# ESSAY 8: SKI PATROL, LIFEGUARD

One day you will read in the National Geographic of a faraway land with no smelly bad traffic. In those green-pastured mountains of Fotta-fa-Zee everybody feels fine at a hundred and three 'cause the air that they breathe is potassium-free and because they chew nuts from the Tutt-a-Tutt Tree. This gives strength to their teeth, it gives length to their hair, and they live without doctors, with nary a care.

—Dr. Seuss, You're Only Old Once

Unfortunately for those of us inhabiting the non-Seussian world, this scenario is about as likely as encountering elephants perched on bird eggs or small furry orators standing atop tree stumps. The book goes on to describe treatment of a type that is seen all too often in our world of doctors. The hapless patient's experience in the clinic is, unfortunately, one that I have shared; it is in fact a driving force behind my motivation to become a physician. My experiences as a child have been instrumental in my current direction: I would like to become the pediatrician I never had. On numerous occasions I was ignored by my family physician simply because I was a child. I was obviously unaware of my body, or at least unable to express myself, since I was less than 5 feet tall. When I walked into the office with my mother, he asked her how I felt, without ever sparing a glance for me (to which my mother generally replied, "Why don't you ask her?"). On those rare occasions on which he did deign to speak to me, it was to remind me of the sunny Saturday on which I was born and the picnic he had to leave because of my imminent arrival. As I grew older and began visiting the office without my parents, he seemed at a loss—what to say to this person who was not yet of a respectable age? He soon settled on, "How are your parents? I still remember that Saturday...." This was, and continues to be, extremely frustrating. Because of my love of and interest in a future career with children, I have sought work with them in several capacities. I have taught them, both as swimming and skiing instructor. I have guided, watched, and played with them as a summer employee at a daycare facility. I have learned much in the process about communicating with them. Time and again, my experience has shown me that, while they are in no way miniature adults, children most certainly are thinking human beings and deserve to be treated as such, although always on a level appropriate to their age.

Outside of my frustrations in the doctor's office, I have found other factors pointing me toward a career in medicine. As I pursued interests in athletics I found ways, sometimes rather unexpectedly, that medicine could take a part. I moved on from teaching skiing to become a volunteer member of the National Ski Patrol. In this way I was able to administer emergency medicine in a setting available to me as an avid skier and a student. I also worked for several summers as a lifeguard. I never really considered, however, that my training would prove so beneficial in my other leisure activities. One afternoon I was out horseback riding with my sister, who is also trained in first aid, when a person came running up the bridle trail. An elderly Parkinson's patient had fallen off a dam, and was gravely injured and in need of immediate aid. I had always assumed that my first real experience with CPR would be more sterile, using a mask and rubber gloves, not riding gloves, to protect me from blood-borne viruses. But this was as messy as it was real, and none of my training had quite prepared me for what I would experience: the exhilaration and single-minded determination to restore life to this person upon whom I had never before laid eyes. Unfortunately, the afternoon did not end as we might have hoped; we were unable to resuscitate him. But the energy and spirit of teamwork surrounding those of us laboring to reclaim this man's life as we waited and waited for an ambulance to arrive were so strong as to be tangible, and called me as nothing ever had before. A heretofore nebulous inclination had become a decision: I wanted to get into this business of shaping lives, but on an extended basis during which I could get to know my patients and help them to maintain and restore their health over time, instead of only intervening when a crisis such as this occurred.

So I have spent my time, playing and singing, traveling and studying those topics that I'm interested in and that will help to shape the person who I am in the process of becoming. There hasn't been nearly enough time for everything I would love to do, but I have found, or more accurately made, time for as much as possible, with the knowledge that there is always more to learn, more to experience. Outside of academics, my major commitment is music, and through my playing and singing, I have been able to visit parts of the country and of the world that I would not otherwise have seen. I have been able to touch the lives of others and bring them joy as I myself have found joy in the dedication to a pursuit and the practice of a skill, not done by rote, but truly performed. This same dedication and love of learning will be invaluable to me as a physician, as will the many experiences which will help me to be more than merely a competent automaton or one of Seuss's "Oglers" who "silently, grimly [ogles] away" at patients, but a vibrant and caring physician. As I can hardly foresee a National Geographic description of a place in which we can live without doctors, I can only strive to be one of those doctors with whom we not only can but also want to live.

## Student Comments

"I actually sat down one afternoon to write the essay; I hate lingering over things for too long. I have something of a history of quoting Dr. Seuss in essays, and my sister bet me that I wouldn't do it this time, so I did. I figured anywhere too uptight to not appreciate a very relevant reference was not somewhere I was interested in going."

## ESSAY 9: COUNSELOR/TEACHER FOR REFUGEE YOUTH PROGRAM AND EMOTIONALLY DISTURBED CHILDREN'S CAMP

Roasting marshmallows on chopsticks over a gas grill, I looked back on how much my relationship with M. had deepened over the 2 years that we had known each other. M., a 13-year-old refugee from Vietnam, had been one of my summer students in the Boston Refugee Youth Enrichment (BRYE) program. On this May night, the two of us were going on a camping trip in M.'s backyard. M. was very well prepared for our adventure: a poster bearing the stern admonition "KEEP AWAY" protected a tent packed with flashlights, pillows, board games, and peanut butter and cheese crackers. These careful arrangements reflected M.'s excitement about the overnight that we were braving together; I shared this excitement, and realized how fortunate I was to be spending this night with my student and close friend.

Certainly, M. would not have been excited at the prospect of spending an overnight together when he entered my class 2 years earlier. M. had had behavioral problems during past summers in BRYE, and the BRYE program directors placed him in my class because of my experience Camp R., a camp for emotionally disturbed children. Indeed, M.'s behavior was less than exemplary on the first day of BRYE, and I remember feeling daunted by the challenge of fostering respect between us. Yet somehow, between that first crazy day of BRYE Summer and the night of our camping trip 2 years later, M. and I had moved beyond the guarded relationship of teacher and class troublemaker; we had become very special friends who trusted each other enough to face together the urban wilderness of Dorchester, Massachusetts.

I am not exactly sure how this change occurred; I often find it difficult to identify specific events that have shaped my relationships with M. and others to whom I have grown close through my work with BRYE and Camp R. However, I remember particularly well staying up one night with C., an 8-year-old boy in my bunk at Camp R., after he had been terribly frightened by a nightmare in which spiders were devouring him. I gave C. my high school gym uniform to wear, suggesting that it's ugly, bright orange color might deter spiders with their sensitive compound eyes. Then I sat on his bed and guarded him from spiders until he was able to fall asleep again.

More recently this past February, I had the opportunity to celebrate Tet, the Vietnamese New Year, with the family of B., one of my students from last summer. B.'s family had been well off before the Communist government took away all that they owned with the victory of North Vietnam over the South in 1975. After the father's imprisonment in a reeducation camp for his ties to the South Vietnamese military, the family came to the United States. Soon after their arrival, their new home burned down, exacerbating the hardships that they faced in this country. Nevertheless, eating, talking, and laughing with B. and his sisters, mother, father, and grandmother, I was greatly moved by the strength and resilience that had emerged from this family's love for one another, and deeply honored that they were willing to share this important holiday with me.

These relationships that I have had with M., C., B.'s family, and others have been very meaningful because we have established genuine, mutual trust. C. could feel safe in the knowledge that I would stay by his bed as long as he needed and I treasured his honesty in sharing his feelings with me. B.'s family recognized the sincerity of my respect for them, just as I was comfortable knowing that their affection and respect for me were genuine as well. Such trust, I believe, is the foundation of the relationships I have formed over the past 4 years, and has fostered a closeness that has impacted my life very deeply. Moreover, the importance of trust in the friendships I have had with others has significantly influenced the expectations, goals, and dreams that I have for myself today, including my aspirations for a career in medicine.

My hopes to become a physician were not always motivated by this desire to grow from and give to trusting relationships with others. Since childhood, I have wanted to be a doctor, and it was a sincere fascination with life that first sparked my enthusiasm for medicine. Nothing seemed more amazing to me than the human body, and I thought that I would be fortunate if I could dedicate my life to so challenging and interesting a study. As a child I was eager to understand how the body fends off illness and to explore the fate of food after it is eaten; now I hope to grasp the answers to these and other questions well enough that I can confront successfully many of the challenges that I will face as a doctor.

The people with whom I have shared myself, however, have shown me that being a doctor means more than making a correct diagnosis and applying an appropriate treatment. To me, being a doctor means fostering trust between myself and my patients, so that we can enjoy mutual confidence as we enrich our own lives through shared experiences. It also means establishing trust with my peers. The friendships that I have made with other counselors have been some of the best aspects of my experiences with BRYE and Camp R. Two of my closest friends, T., a year older than I, and S., a year younger, have played especially important roles in my personal growth over the past few years. None of us knew right away the significance that working with Dorchester's Vietnamese refugee community would hold for us. However, through sharing our insights into the challenges, failures, and successes we experienced, as well as our passion for the work we were doing, each of us grew and learned more together than any one of us could have done on our own. Similarly, given the demands of becoming a good doctor, I believe that many of my colleagues will share a passion for medicine akin to Steve and Theresa's passion for BRYE.

I very much hope to be a part of such a community of men and women who, through facing together the challenges and hardships of being physicians, enrich each other's lives just as they enrich the lives of the patients to whom they have dedicated themselves.

Thus, after my experiences over the past 4 years with BRYE and Camp R., I believe that my commitment to the medical profession will be a commitment, above all else, to the children, women, and men whom I serve, as well as to the men and women with whom I serve. Although I realize that I cannot become lifelong friends with everyone I meet, I hope that the comfort we feel in our mutual trust and respect will make some difference in our lives. Indeed, I am sometimes daunted by the difficulty I will inevitably face in encouraging others to place their trust in me as I place my trust in them, for I will not always be able to fulfill the needs of everyone whom I serve. Nevertheless, I am eager to make this commitment, for no experiences in my life have been as happy or gratifying as those that I have shared intimately with others. If, as a doctor, I can continue giving to, learning from, and sharing with others as I have as a counselor and teacher over the past 4 years, I believe that my life will be a fulfilling one; it is to this end that I hope to dedicate myself. Reminiscing about how M. pulled the browned marshmallow from his chopstick, I am thankful to my campers and students, their families, and my friends for helping me to affirm that this is the path I wish my life to follow.

## Student Comments

"I found that having a somewhat nonstandard essay helped a great deal in interviews. In almost all of my interviews I was able to discuss the experiences described in my essay in some depth. This way, I was walking on familiar ground and was not floored by a lot of tricky questions. That is, an interesting personal statement can promote a good discussion during interview."

## ESSAY 10: ENVIRONMENTAL STUDY IN AFRICA, COMMUNITY SERVICE, LITERACY VOLUNTEER

"Why on Earth do you want to study in Africa?" is a question I remember being asked frequently before I went to Kenya for the Dartmouth College Environmental Studies Program. At the time, I thought the question was absurd—I could not understand why anyone would not jump at the opportunity to live among and learn about such diverse and exciting peoples. However, after my 3 months of study throughout Kenya, I realized that not everyone could endure, much less enjoy, the experiences I had. For some people, the pit latrines, absence of running water, malarial mosquitoes, and mud-dung huts would have defined the experience. For me, it was so much more: my time in Kenya was shaped by the Samburu pastoralists that shared their homes with us for a week, by the wild animals that we studied for hours on end, by the Kamba agriculturists that gave us a glimpse of their lifestyle over a weekend homestay, and by my Luo family in Nairobi. Indeed, my sojourns in Kenya would not have been enjoyed by everyone. But they were the profoundly educational and humanitarian experiences on which I thrive.

A career in medicine appears to be a lot like studying in Kenya. It is challenging, intense, filled with hard work, and extremely rewarding—but not for everyone. Many people cannot see beyond the years of demanding course work, sleep deprivation, and long work hours that are associated with the study and practice of medicine. Although these are realities of a physician's life, they are not what define it for me. A career as a physician excites me because it would allow me to further understand the fascinating science that dictates human life, and more importantly, it would allow me to work closely with people, while trying to understand and alleviate their suffering. My love for learning and passion for helping people drove me to Kenya, and they also fuel my desire to become a physician.

My first encounter with medical science was as a "Women in Science" Intern in the Norris Cotton Cancer Center of the Dartmouth-Hitchcock Medical Center. I worked in the radiobiology lab of Dr. J., and was given the task of designing and carrying out experiments to measure the absorption and scattering coefficients of laser light in tissue simulating media, for use in the development of photodynamic therapy (PDT) as a cancer treatment. The project was so exciting to me that it developed into a full-time summer position, which culminated in my contribution to a scientific paper, currently being reviewed by several journals for publication. My interest in the projects of Dr. J.'s laboratory was so substantial that I continued to work with her after the completion of the PDT project for over a year. Specifically, I assisted with experiments to correlate the rate of blood flow and the partial pressure of oxygen in tumors. My work resulted in a contribution to another abstract, submitted to the Regional Conference on Cancer Research at the UVM Cancer Center in Burlington, Vermont.

In addition to my enthusiasm for science, I have a deep-rooted interest in art history. My curiosity about the subject was sparked in high school;

and by the time I graduated, it had become one of my favorite subjects. My interest continued through college and culminated in 3 months of study in Florence, Italy, with the Dartmouth college Art History Program. I hope to continue my study of art history throughout my life. Artistic interpretation is a good balance for data analysis and scientific exploration; it provides insight into an entirely different way of viewing the world.

However, both my research experiences and my study of art have left me devoid of the satisfaction of helping people that I have felt throughout high school and college, working directly with several community service organizations. When I was 15, I volunteered at a local hospital. Although I had few responsibilities, it was the first time I had interacted with patients. The satisfaction I derived from assisting these people solidified my desire to help others. That same summer, I traveled with several other students to Middlebury, Vermont to repair a homeless shelter. Later in high school, I became a member of Literacy Volunteers of America and tutored adult students in a local adult education center. Throughout my college career, I have been involved with Dartmouth's Students Fighting Hunger chapter. Few things in my college career have been as rewarding as working to help feed the people of the Upper Valley region through community-awareness programs, fund-raising projects, and direct assistance in soup kitchens. Seeking to learn about the union of science and compassion in medical practice, I am spending part of this summer as a Student Observer in the Memorial Sloan-Kettering Cancer Center, Department of Thoracic Surgery. One of my highest priorities is to remain involved in humanitarian assistance throughout my life. The medical field would provide an ideal setting for me to fulfill this goal.

A career as a physician would unite my excitement for learning and my desire for helping others into a distinct whole. My life so far has been filled with many diverse experiences, teaching me much about both my own interest and the way in which I can best serve humanity, I look forward to integrating my interests and talents into a 4-year medical education, and a lifelong medical career.

## Orphanage Volunteer in Brazil

When I entered Dartmouth College in 1987, I was amazed by the large number of students already labeled as "premeds." I wondered how those students were able to decide with such certainty that they wanted to study medicine, and I imagined that they all must have known from a very early age that they would one day be great doctors. I had no such inklings, and if asked as a child what I wanted to be when I grew up, I would have said that I wanted to be an Olympic skier or soccer player. While in high school, my achievement in various science courses prompted several friends and teachers to ask if I was interested in becoming a doctor. My negative response to their queries was largely based on my mistaken notion that since I didn't grow up knowing I wanted to be a doctor, I probably wasn't cut out for a career in medicine. I realize now that the decision to pursue a career in medicine must be based on much more than an instinctively positive feeling about becoming a doctor. I now know that making the decision to study medicine requires careful examination of one's reasons for wanting to be a doctor, an understanding of the rigors of medical training and the demanding nature of the profession, and perhaps most importantly, the maturity to make the great commitment that is necessary in order to achieve the goal of becoming an excellent physician.

People often ask me when I decided that I wanted to be a doctor. My response to that seemingly straightforward question is not a simple one since several years elapsed from the time that I initially became interested in medicine until I decided to apply to medical school. My job volunteering in an orphanage in Brazil during my sophomore year in college was extremely influential in shaping my current goals. At the orphanage, I lived with 30 young girls and 4 Portuguese-speaking, Japanese nuns in the countryside, several hours by car from Sao Paulo. My daily chores included everything from caring for babies and teaching the older girls English to harvesting vegetable crops before they were destroyed by summer floods and even fishing in the hope of adding an extra source of protein to our diets. While helping out at the orphanage and getting to know the children was a unique and exciting experience, I was somewhat frustrated by the fact that I didn't have any specific skill or service to offer the people I met in Brazil. I considered what type of work I would like to do if I ever returned to Brazil or another developing country, and I began to think about how rewarding it would be to be a doctor in such a place where the need for even basic health care services was dire. Pursuing a career in medicine seemed like an ideal way to balance both my desire to work with disadvantaged people either abroad or at home and my desire to work in a dynamic, intellectually challenging field. However, I hesitated to commit myself to the difficult and time-consuming goal of becoming a doctor, and I wondered whether my interest in medicine would endure when I returned to college or whether it was a transient manifestation of idealism engendered by my experience working with the poor in Brazil. As it turned out, thoughts of becoming a doctor never left me after living in Brazil, and although I didn't immediately commit myself to the idea of going to medical school, I decided to keep my options open by exploring some biology courses when I returned to Dartmouth.

I missed the sense of satisfaction that I had experienced while working with the children in Brazil when I began working for a management consulting firm after I graduated from college. Although I enjoyed the problem-solving nature of consulting, my interest in improving the business practices of client companies was limited. I worked hard and performed well while in consulting, but I longed for a sense of accomplishment greater than that which I was able to realize while working in business. I began to consider returning to school to complete my medical school prerequisite courses, and I found that my perspective regarding the great commitment associated with a medical career had changed since college as a result of my experience working in business. I was excited rather than daunted when I thought about the challenges I would encounter in medical school and throughout my medical career because I had gained a new understanding of the importance of pursuing a career that I would find both intellectually stimulating and personally rewarding.

I returned to school after working in consulting for almost a year. While I enjoyed my prerequisite science courses this past year, it was my experience volunteering as a patient history taker and a lab assistant at the Free Medical Clinic of Cleveland that truly confirmed my desire to be a doctor. As a history taker, I met with each patient before he or she was seen by a doctor, and I was responsible for recording each patient's relevant past history, current symptoms, and vital signs. Many of the people I interviewed were teenagers or young adults with health problems related to their sexual activity. After observing other history takers and conducting interviews, myself, I gained confidence in my ability to ask pertinent questions based on preliminary information offered by the frequently scared or embarrassed patients, and I found that I was able to put patients at ease in situations that had the potential to be very uncomfortable for them. Working in the medical lab at the Clinic complemented my history-taking experience. I observed which tests doctors ordered based on the different symptoms presented by patients, I conducted some of the lab tests myself, and I observed the doctors interpret the test results that helped them make their diagnoses. I learned a great deal while working at the Clinic, and I left Cleveland feeling satisfied that I had contributed something to the community in which I had lived and looking forward to medical school more than ever.

My experiences in taking premedical courses, volunteering at the Cleveland Free Clinic, and working with nontraditional, premedical students like myself at Harvard Summer School have all served to convince me that I want to be a practicing physician. I needed time after college to reach that conclusion, and I believe that I will be a better medical student, and hopefully a better doctor, as a result of my varied experiences and careful questioning of my motivations for wanting to become a doctor. I am currently anticipating the start of my new job working as a research assistant in the intensive care unit at Boston Children's Hospital, and I am confident that working at Children's Hospital will further strengthen my desire to pursue a career in medicine.

## Student Comments

"I worked hard on my essay to explain my decision to leave a job in consulting and to pursue a career in medicine. I think it's important for 'nontraditional' applicants to give the chronology of the various things they have done, but more importantly to explain their motivation to leave behind other interesting opportunities and to accept the challenge of becoming a physician. Also, it is so important to be honest since one will be asked many times about the personal statement when interviewing, and it's painfully obvious when a student exaggerates or is overly dramatic when recounting their experiences (I served on the Harvard Med admissions committee)."

# ESSAY 11: CAREER SWITCHER FROM MARKETING MANAGEMENT

I was not in control of my life and I was miserable. Forced by my parents' unwillingness to pay for my education, I worked as a branch manager for a marketing corporation. From April to September, I spent 12 to 14 hours at work each day, doing everything possible to make enough money to return to school the following year. Amid the hard work, I lost track of who I was and what I wanted in life. I lost touch with my friends and the people that I cared about.

In spite of this, the experience was worthwhile. As a manager in charge of 46 people, I learned valuable skills of communication and personal interaction which related to my goal of working in the medical profession. Every day, I had the opportunity to interview several new people, to talk to them, and get to know a little about them. In addition, through functions in and out of the office, I became very close with the core of my sales force. Not only did I teach them how to sell our product, but also listened to their personal problems and gave them advice. As a result, I had the pleasure of receiving a letter from one of my salespersons at the end of the summer thanking me for the skills that she had learned and the self-confidence that she had gained.

Later that year, however, I decided to begin to regain control of my life. Although I realized that it would increase financial pressures, I chose to stop working for the marketing corporation and prepare more directly for a career in medicine. I accepted a job in a laboratory at the University of Pennsylvania School of Medicine in order to broaden my experience and ensure that I was choosing the right profession.

In high school, I had experience dealing directly with patients. I assisted the athletic trainer, taping players, treating injuries, and making diagnoses. The experience was enjoyable because I learned a great deal about sports medicine, including anatomy and muscle function. It also showed me the importance of teamwork in medicine. Having been an athlete, I recognized the power of teamwork on the field. Yet, I had been unaware of the cooperation needed in the training room. The most worthwhile aspect of the experience, however, was the trust and respect that the players showed toward me. After I became comfortable working by myself, I could sense that they felt secure when I treated them.

Research was new to me, yet I was impressed by the intellectual challenges that it presented. I appreciated the systematic approach and planning that were required to solve problems and direct research. I liked the attention to detail that was needed to be successful. I enjoyed the atmosphere of the laboratory and the cooperative spirit of the researchers. Most of all, however, I was attracted by the idea that I could have impact on many lives by conducting research.

The research experience that I have had, combined with my sister's recent cancer diagnosis and therapy, changed my view on my future in medicine. Previously, I had planned to work only in the clinic, so that I could have personal contact with patients. Now, I also feel a responsibility to contribute to the advancement of medical science. I intend to perform research so that others may avoid hardships like the one that my sister has undergone during the past year.

Focused on my career goal, I have retaken control of my life. I have decided what I want to do and who I want to be. I have found a career that will balance my intellectual curiosity with my longing for personal interaction. I have found a career that will engage my interests and will be fulfilling for me.

# ESSAY 12: COMMUNITY HEALTH VOLUNTEER IN HAITI, INTERNATIONAL DEVELOPMENT, AND PUBLIC HEALTH BACKGROUND

"Dawn, do you believe in las brujas?" In witches?! I was just concluding a workshop on diarrhea and dehydration with a group of community health workers. In the border region between the Dominican Republic and Haiti, it is commonly believed that the symptoms of dehydration are a result of children being "sucked by witches." So I diplomatically answered that although where I grew up people don't tend to believe in witches, undeniably there are places where individuals are more strongly influenced by the powers of magic. Apparently encouraged by my response, the women—who I trained and supervised as part of a mother-infant health program—proceeded to recount numerous tales of children's lives being saved by curanderos, or witch doctors, after having been "sucked."

In my mind, I was scrambling for a way to salvage our discussion of hygiene and oral rehydration. After listening carefully to their stories, I pointed out that despite the wide variety of rituals, prayers, and herbs used to free the victim of witches, each of the "cures" they described involved the administration of liquids. They were soon deciding that whether a mother chooses to believe that her child has been affected by witches or by bacteria, it is always important to rehydrate the child. We concluded the meeting saying that when appropriate, properly prepared oral rehydration salts could be utilized as "anti-witch" treatment.

The complexity of human health has led me to the study of medicine. At the time of that training, my background included a degree in international development and experience working on community health programs in several countries. I expected that my next academic pursuit would be a master's in public health. However, along with increased exposure to the field, came the realization that I wanted more.

I wanted to be able to do more. While aware of the enormous value of health instruction and disease prevention, I found myself often feeling frustrated with the limitations of what I had to offer. People benefit from education and training, but at times they also need medicines and treatment. My efforts to help people improve their quality of life could be enhanced by expanding my capabilities. The study of medicine would greatly increase the impact that I could have on people's health.

I also wanted to know and understand more. Less altruistic than a desire to help others—yet an equally powerful motivating force in my life—is my love of learning. I have always found that for work to be truly satisfying to me, it must be intellectually stimulating. To conduct an effective health education campaign, one must learn to communicate information in a simplistic fashion, yet my own questions about health issues were increasingly complex. I wasn't content just knowing that diarrhea leads to dehydration; I was wondering how and why and what could be done to treat it and how does that work? With minimal preparation in the sciences, the challenge of entering a new academic field was enticing. Medical knowledge would afford me a much broader perspective on human health.

If both the physiology of dehydration and the belief that a child is being "sucked by witches" can be understood, then a person's health needs will be more effectively met. I now intend to study both medicine and public health, since I feel that an interdisciplinary approach is best suited for confronting multifaceted health problems.

## Student Comments

"It took me a few months to write and revise the essay. I gave it to lots of people—both knowledgeable of the med school application process and not—to read and criticize. I think that my essay was a very significant part of my application, since in all of my interviews the story I related was a prominent topic of conversation. I know people have been hearing this since they applied to college, but the first sentence is crucial—it's the one chance to grab the attention of an admissions officer who may be reading thousands of essays. Personally, I also like to start out essays with an anecdote."

# ESSAY 13: CAREER SWITCHER FROM VETERINARIAN TECHNICIAN, EMERGENCY MEDICAL TECHNICIAN, PARENTS' INFLUENCE

She dropped the box on the table and left the room because she didn't want to watch. I could understand her feelings: many of our clients at the veterinary clinic chose not to observe the distressing moment when life slipped away from their pet. Still, I always felt for the animals whose owners couldn't face the reality of the decision they'd made, animals who would die surrounded by relative strangers.

As I waited for the veterinarian to come perform the euthanasia, I stroked the dehydrated cat's bony back. She lay still, tired from fighting the sickness. My petting her seemed a necessity: the only way to provide one final pleasure for this old animal. She barely responded, maybe a slight twitch of the whiskers. But then, just before the vet stepped into the room, my little patient started to purr. It began softly but grew to a warm rumble, filling the room with the sound of a cat's contentedness. I had, happily, made this cat as comfortable as was possible. She kept on purring even as I held her and the doctor injected the thick pink solution into her vein. The sound faded quietly as her body went limp in my arms.

As a veterinary technician, I don't think I could have asked for a better introduction to the power of medicine. At the clinic I experienced first-hand the day-to-day life of medical practice. We treated outpatient and boarding animals who were essentially healthy: administering vaccines, drawing blood, giving daily medications, and offering general medical advice. I performed lab tests and maintain hospital supplies. We also cared for animals whose conditions were critical: I noted their progress, reported to the doctor, and carried out his orders for treatment.

Therapies included special feeding, intravenous or subcutaneous fluid administration, and medications of all kinds. This intensive care afforded me the chance to observe diagnostic techniques and the decisions for treatments that were based on the diagnoses. I also assisted during surgery, monitoring the vital signs of the patient using only a stethoscope, the air bag, and my intuition for what was normal. I performed the pre- and post-operative duties and any treatments that were more easily done while the animals were sedated, such as thorough dental cleaning. I was therefore able to see the excitement of surgery and the satisfaction of using one's hands to directly heal a body.

Over those 2 years, I decided that I wanted to apply to medical school rather than veterinary school. I gradually found myself feeling out of touch with a large part of humanity. I realized that the pleasure of healing would be greater for me if the patients were people. This realization has been affirmed in my recent experiences shadowing doctors and training as a medical assistant. I feel there are greater challenges involved in caring for human beings: treatment of critical illness in animals halts before human care does, since euthanasia is a readily available option for veterinarians. Human medicine therefore goes beyond most animal care, delving deeper to fight disease. In addition, there is a psychological dimension to human medicine that attracts me. Of course, interaction with patients is richer; I value and hope to encourage the contributions that patients make to their own well-being and health care.

The true causes of healing and the role of the mind in restoring and maintaining the body are subjects that I find extremely compelling.

My training and experiences with medicine have contributed to how I envision myself practicing it. I greatly enjoyed the diversity of medicine practiced at the vet clinic; for this and other reasons I lean toward primary care or emergency medicine. In order to explore the latter option I am pursuing certification as an Emergency Medical Technician. I also appreciate the individual nature of service provided by a small, modest clinic, and would like to provide such personal care for the people I treat. I look forward to getting to know my patients as well as we at the clinic knew our clients and their pets.

I realize in retrospect that as a young girl I always assumed I would be a doctor. My father was a psychiatrist, and my mother entered medical school when I entered kindergarten. My mother provides a role model I still look to for guidance. Throughout my high school years and into my first year at college, I pursued activities in the medical sciences, such as advanced courses and a summer research assistant job at N.I.H. Although I began college as a premedical student, the wider options presented to me at school made me eager to explore other disciplines. I turned away from science during my undergraduate years, but am confident that my Swarthmore education will be invaluable in my development as a well-rounded physician. My experiences in medicine, healing the sick, comforting the ill and dying, and even the routine aspects of the work, hold a power for me that I cannot ignore. Since arriving at this decision and acting on it, I feel that I have come full circle. I have ended up in many ways where I began, but with far more experience. This is exactly where I want to be.

## Student Comments

"I don't think my essay was crucial in my acceptance, as my MCAT scores were very good, and my grades good. As well, I had worked and lived a while before applying, which broadened my experiences.

One tip on applying in general: Talk to 3rd and 4th years, and listen to what they say. They know more about medical school in general, and theirs in particular. Also, the clinical years really are more important than years 1 and 2. Look at what the clinical experience will be like in judging which school you want."

# ESSAY 14: TENNIS

The car swerved to the left. A sudden impact forced me out of my sitting position in the back of the station wagon. Everything became still as I heard the uneasy voice of my mother's friend in the driver's seat: "Mrs. K., Mrs. K.!" She became frantic and started crying, muttering phrases that I did not understand. What I did know was that my mother was not answering her cries. I sat and stared at the back of the passenger's seat of the car, trying to make sense of what was happening. I was 7 and the only thing I knew was that something was wrong. I did not cry; I did not call out to my mom. I sat frozen, listening intently for my mother's voice, watching my mom's friend plead through tears, and wondering why she was not doing anything to help her. A short while later, ambulances arrived. After someone helped me out of the car, I tried to get to my mom. The paramedics would not let me near her, but I saw her with her head tilted back into the seat and groaning softly. Her eyelids were shut but the shape and wrinkles of her face told me that she was in immense pain.

My mother broke her right arm in the accident, leaving her unable to care of my 7-month-old sister. At first seeing my mother so helpless was as distressing as my fear during the accident. During the next several months, I discovered that the act of helping allayed my fears. Even now my mother's face glows with affection each time she recalls how at the age of 7, I helped bathe, feed, and change the diapers of my baby sister. The desire to help and care for my mom and my sister was instinctive; she never needed to ask.

Driven by this instinct, the urge to learn through helping has remained strong. In high school I helped cook and serve meals in a soup kitchen on Sundays. I also devoted my time to the E.R. of Lake West Hospital. Upon graduating, I worked in the pediatric I.C.U. of the Cleveland Clinic. Since then, I have also volunteered at the Massachusetts General Hospital. All of these opportunities have been invaluable, but the most rewarding has been my role as a Big Sister for an 8-year-old girl through the United Way Big Sister Association. Y. emigrated with her family from Hong Kong only 1 year ago. Her family, lacking both the financial resources and the knowledge of English, is rarely able to take her out of Chinatown and introduce her to her new environment. In spite of our language barrier, Y. and I have become fast friends through 6-hour outings every Saturday. From patiently teaching her "Mary Had a Little Lamb" on the piano to drawing pictures to explain why "my daddy and mommy" do not live in my dorm room, I truly enjoy every moment with her. What makes this volunteer job so much more meaningful than the others is that it does not end at the end of my shift. It means I can come back to my dorm room after a tiring day of classes, play back my answering machine, and hear her sweet voice sing a Chinese lullaby for me. It means that this is not a volunteer job: she gives just as much to me as I give to her.

My eagerness to care for others coupled with my father's influence as a physician developed my interest in health care through biomedical research. Specifically, I have worked independently on two projects. I mastered cell culture techniques to study the effects of nerve and epidermal growth factors on amyloid precursor protein ectodomain secretion in rat pheochromocytoma cells (applied to Alzheimer's disease). I was fortunate enough to obtain favorable results, which are in the process of being published. My current project is analyzing the effects of leptin, the protein product of the obesity gene, on insulin regulation (applied to diabetes). I am responsible for conducting and quantifying experiments in pancreatic beta cell lines, as well as assaying insulin, corticosteroid, and glucose levels of experiments done in vivo. My enjoyment of laboratory research stems from two levels. First, being directly involved in the process of uncovering new knowledge, rather than simply absorbing knowledge uncovered by others is exhilarating. Second, the road of many hours of hard work and repetition resolving in a slow but stimulating process is familiar and encouraging—I have traveled this same road by playing 10 years of competitive tennis.

I realize that succeeding in medicine requires more than a desire to help others. A career in medicine demands great perseverance and dedication to both scientific and humanistic knowledge. I believe I have acquired these characteristics through my academic, extracurricular, and research experiences. These qualities in addition to my concern for others will enable me to care for my future patients with sensitivity and understanding. The once bewildered 7-year-old at the scene of an accident now has the skills and maturity to do more than change diapers; she aspires to read the film of the broken humerus or to set the cast someday soon.

## Student Comments

"My advice would be to try to include things that do NOT show up elsewhere on your application that you feel might be relevant. When starting out, make a list of jobs/personal qualities/events that you would like to include and among those, see if you can connect them into a 'theme' for your essay."